AF283926

Ways to Quit Drinking

A Sober Curious Book on How to Control
Alcohol for Better Health, Self-Esteem
and Mental Clarity

Michelle Matthews and Tony Matthews

© Copyright 2024 - All rights reserved.

The content contained within this book may not be reproduced, duplicated or transmitted without direct written permission from the authors or the publisher.

Under no circumstances will any blame or legal responsibility be held against the publisher, or authors, for any damages, reparation, or monetary loss due to the information contained within this book, either directly or indirectly.

Legal Notice:

This book is copyright protected. It is only for personal use. You cannot amend, distribute, sell, use, quote or paraphrase any part, or the content within this book, without the consent of the authors or publisher.

Disclaimer Notice:

Please note the information contained within this document is for educational and entertainment purposes only. All effort has been executed to present accurate, up to date, reliable, complete information. No warranties of any kind are declared or implied. Readers acknowledge that the authors are not engaged in the rendering of legal, financial, medical or professional advice. The content within this book has been derived from various sources. Please consult a licensed professional before attempting any techniques outlined in this book.

By reading this document, the reader agrees that under no circumstances are the authors responsible for any losses, direct or indirect, that are incurred as a result of the use of the information contained within this document, including, but not limited to, errors, omissions, or inaccuracies.

Table of Contents

Preface, aka Do We Really Need Another Book on Quitting Drinking?

As I sit here on this balmy summer evening, sipping my favourite sparkling water with a big squeeze of fresh lemon, I'm reflecting on the path that brought my husband Tony and me to where we are today. We're your typical middle-aged couple, living in the suburbs, focused on our careers and family. To the outside world, everything probably seems normal – almost boringly so.

But behind our metaphorical white picket fence, we've contended with an issue familiar to millions yet rarely openly discussed – dependence on alcohol. You'd never have guessed it if you ran into me strolling our black Labrador around the block on weekends or caught Tony cheerfully pottering in the garden. By all appearances, we seemed to have it together.

However, for over a decade, we struggled largely in silence with drinking more than we knew was wise. It crept up on us, as harmless weekend unwinding shifted into daily reflex. At first, we justified it as simply blowing off steam, a reward after long days managing hectic careers and rambunctious kids.

But over time, our drinking habits became less about relaxation and enjoyment and more about dependence. I began planning my days around that first evening drink, only feeling relief as I poured my second or third glass of wine each night. Tony would observe me trying to abstain – or at least moderate – at times and hear me lament that I needed to not drink so much, so often. I know he secretly hoped I would not insist he also endeavour to drink less. So, we both gave in to the nagging voices convincing ourselves it was harmless to have a 'cheers and a kiss' and drink wine together in the evenings. After all, most people drink, don't they? This is Australia. It's what we do.

We hid it well, but the signs were there. Mornings spent recovering from headaches and exhaustion from poor sleep. Tasks not done, due to regularly falling asleep on the sofa, and the resulting increasing tension between us over small issues. Discomfort at social events, trying to consume drinks at double the rate that everyone else seemed to need to, without them noticing that's what I was doing. My frequent attempts to cut back – a 'dry' January here or there – ultimately collapsing. All while maintaining appearances as a doting school mum and happy self-employed small business owner.

It was a merry-go-round we couldn't seem to stop. The headaches, weight gain and feelings of shame mounted, until suddenly – I stepped off the ride. No fanfare or rock bottom moment. After a particular family birthday celebration, I simply felt so incredibly frustrated at the sheer daily struggle of trying to moderate and control my intake that – literally – I threw my hands in the air and said, 'That's it', and, 'I'm not drinking for 12 months'. After three short weeks, the relief was so very great, and the feelings of elation at having conquered the beast so enormous, I decided that was it – for good. I made the decision to live alcohol-free. Observing this, Tony joined me. I didn't ask him or tell him to. We didn't even discuss it. We just knew.

It hasn't always been easy, but, armed with analytical minds and a burgeoning passion for living a long and healthy life, we pieced together a personalised plan incorporating the physical, mental and emotional tools needed to maintain an alcohol-free lifestyle. Meanwhile, we both pursued coaching certifications focused specifically on cultivating healthier relationships with our emotions and the plethora of distractions we as human beings employ to avoid dealing with them, with Tony going on to successfully coach many individuals battling with similar challenges to those we knew only too well.

Though our expertise lies in applying scientific rigour to our research and therapeutic principles to our coaching, our authority comes from lived experience. We intimately understand the struggle because we've been there – concealing how many 'refills' we're having, dropping wine bottles carefully into the bin so we don't sound like a recycling facility to the neighbours, having a drink or two before going out so we don't have to worry about getting enough.

We won't pretend to have all the answers or a one-size-fits-all solution. Everyone has a unique relationship with alcohol influenced by countless emotional, genetic and environmental variables. As certified coaches rather than clinicians, we aim to compassionately guide you to interrogate your own relationship, determine your 'why' and define the optimal path forward.

Consider us simply neighbours who happen to have specialised knowledge from walking in similar shoes. We transcended unhealthy drinking by piecing together a bespoke and holistic plan – one we strive to model in this book. We hope our blend of personal narrative and evidence-based solutions helps clarify rather than confuse, encourage rather than discourage.

Mostly, we aim to help anyone trapped in painful drinking cycles realise that there is light beyond the daily hangovers, secrecy and shame. Healing, happiness and genuine human connection await. We should know – we live it each day beyond the white picket fence. (The one the black Labrador escapes from any chance she gets!)

Introduction

If you've picked up this book, chances are you have an uncomfortable relationship with alcohol. Maybe you worry that your nightly wine with dinner has edged into unhealthy territory. Perhaps those bottles are adding up faster than you'd like to admit. Or maybe you've tried cutting back before, only to end up right where you started.

Trust us, we've been there. We know that feeling of dread when the clock strikes five and the pull of 'wine o'clock' takes over. We recognise the denial and frustration when others comment on our drinking, even lightly. We remember all too well those mornings spent struggling through work emails with a pounding head, swearing 'never again'... until the same thing happens tomorrow.

So you wonder — am I overreacting? Is this just normal stress-induced drinking? Or is it possible my alcohol use has crept from casual enjoyment towards dependence?

The truth is, it doesn't really matter where you land on the spectrum. If you feel conflicted enough about your drinking to ponder those questions, if your gut instinct tells you something is off, then this book is for you.

Because here's what we've learned first-hand: Half measures of moderation rarely work long-term once alcohol has its hooks in you. The temporary highs lead to the same low points again and again. And those lows block you from reaching your full potential as a parent, partner, professional or simply a healthy human. And don't we all want to be the best version of ourselves we can be? And live the life of our dreams?

The Benefits Await You

The good news is, there is another way. In this book, we'll share the precise personalised plan that helped us leave damaging drinking habits behind for good. Yes, for good – but we'll get there one step at a time, together.

First, we'll dig into why problem drinking develops in the first place – minus the judgement, but with compassionate understanding and scientific evidence. Next, we'll survey the landscape of liberation options, from traditionally acknowledged alcoholic treatment programs to emerging 'sober curious' movements (no, you do not need to label yourself an 'alcoholic' to change course).

Finally, we'll outline a step-by-step process for cobbling together the physical, mental and emotional building blocks that empower lasting change. This includes everything from nutrition fundamentals to subtle mindset shifts, new coping tools and beyond.

Guiding you along the way are not preachy clinicians or newly sober influencers – but the analytical minds of an engineer and emotions coach who have been where you are. We'll decode complex concepts into applicable tactics. We'll share straight-talk around what worked for us... and what didn't.

Most importantly, we'll help reframe this challenge as an opportunity – not a limitation. With the energy, clarity and purpose you'll gain, imagine the positive ripples you'll create as a partner, parent, friend and passionate soul once freed from alcohol's grip.

This Is Your Path Forward

So, take a deep breath. You've likely worried alone about your drinking for too long – your secret shame in the shadows. Consider this book the sunlight that helps to remove those shadows.

Inside this book lies everything you need to write your next life chapter completely on your own terms – without alcohol hijacking the story. It likely won't happen overnight, but, inch by inch, small daily progress will compound into transformation. Together, word by word, we'll author the story of the person you most want to become – and deserve to be.

This is your path forward. The first step starts now as you turn this page. We can't wait to take it with you.

Chapter 1:

In the Beginning There Was Water... And Then Along Came Alcohol

You've probably heard the phrase 'double-edged sword'. Something that, while offering benefits, can also cause harm. That's alcohol in a nutshell.

In some cultures, it's an integral part of celebrations and social gatherings, yet it's also a cause of numerous health problems and societal issues.

On one hand, moderate consumption of certain types of alcohol, like red wine, is claimed to be associated with heart health benefits.

On the other hand, excessive consumption of alcohol can lead to a myriad of health problems ranging from liver diseases to cancer.

Furthermore, alcohol plays a significant role in our social interactions. It often acts as an icebreaker in social settings and can make people feel more relaxed and sociable.

However, it can also lead to impaired judgement and reckless decisions that might be deeply regretted later.

And let's not forget its economic impact. The alcohol industry contributes significantly to the economy through job creation and tax revenues.

But it also incurs costs related to healthcare, law enforcement and lost productivity due to alcohol-related illnesses and accidents.

Alcohol is truly a double-edged sword. Its effects range from the celebration of life's milestones to the instigator of life-altering health conditions.

It's a social lubricant that can turn into a social liability.

And it's an economic contributor that can become an economic burden.

As we take a closer look into this topic while deciding the place alcohol will have (or not have) in our lives, we'll find that understanding alcohol is not only about knowing its chemical composition or its effects on the body. It's about understanding its complex role in our society and in our lives.

It's about navigating its benefits and harms and making informed decisions about our own consumption.

Because at the end of the day, alcohol is not just a drink. It's a powerful substance that can shape our health, our relationships and our world.

The purpose of this chapter is to tease out the pros and cons of the alcohol phenomenon – inspecting each fact individually. While we are clearly a wee bit biased since we've chosen to not have alcohol as part of our personal diet – we admit that! – we aim to be objective and give both the benefits and downsides of alcohol a fair hearing. Because as mature, worldly types, we're pragmatic enough to acknowledge that we did enjoy many of the 'benefits' of alcohol for a good portion of those years, before the downsides were clearly outweighing the upsides.

But why interrogate the 'pros' and 'cons' so closely?

To effectively solve problems and make informed decisions, we must have access to clear and accurate facts and data. By basing our choices on sound reasoning, thorough research and contemplation, we can move forward confidently, free from doubt.

Let's have a look at the origins and the pros and cons of alcohol in its many guises.

The Origins of Alcohol: Deeply Rooted in Human History

Humans have been brewing and consuming alcohol for thousands of years – evidence exists for fermented drinks dating back to 7000–6600 B.C.E. in ancient China. Around 5000 B.C.E., wine also emerged in ancient Egypt and Mesopotamia. These early societies fermented various fruits, grains and other natural substances to create alcoholic beverages for religious, medicinal and social purposes.

In fact, according to a study published in the *Proceedings of the National Academy of Sciences*, our ancestors may have started drinking alcohol as far back as 10 million years ago when they developed an enzyme that could metabolise ethanol – the type of alcohol found in fermented fruits (Carrigan et al., 2014).

The study suggests that this evolutionary adaptation was crucial for the survival of our primate ancestors, allowing them to consume overripe fruit without getting sick. This discovery implies that our relationship with alcohol is not merely cultural, but biological.

Over centuries, alcohol became deeply intertwined with agriculture, rituals, cuisine and social customs across many cultures. Advances in distillation increased access, unlocking spirits, liqueurs and more. By the 1800s, innovations enabled large-scale beer and liquor production.

Today, alcohol remains inextricably woven with human progress, for better or worse! Billions consume it for purposes ranging from religious rituals to creative pursuits to simple enjoyment. This long, complex relationship reflects alcohol's unique talent to profoundly alter moods, behaviours and cravings. It's almost as if this crafty molecule has tapped into our primal thirst for altered states of consciousness.

And therein lies a problem. Alcohol is here to stay. Yet, for some of us, its presence brings both blessings and burdens.

Alcohol has beguiled humans across our existence, irresistible in its ability to disinhibit and unlock new planes. We return despite sometimes foggy memories of questionable adventures under its influence! As long as we've roamed Earth, we've been unable to resist alcohol's mystical allure. Here's hoping humanity handles responsibly the profound powers within this genie's bottle.

The Pros: Alcohol's Diverse Industrial Applications

Alcohol, including ethanol (or ethyl alcohol), methanol, isopropanol and butanol, demonstrates remarkable versatility and serves invaluable roles across industries, fulfilling numerous critical purposes.

As a disinfectant, alcohol (particularly ethanol and isopropanol) sanitises surfaces, medical equipment and skin, preventing infections and saving lives. Its germ-killing properties as an antiseptic, battling both bacteria and viruses, are essential for health and safety.

By preserving organisms from microbes to cells, alcohol enables scientific advances. It stabilises lab solutions (facilitating scientific progress), protects injectables (medications and vaccines) and substantially lengthens product shelf-life (for example, in cosmetics) through its ability to inhibit the growth of bacteria and fungi.

Alcohol – methanol or ethanol, for instance – can be used for de-icing purposes, such as on planes and vehicle windshields, due to its ability to lower the freezing point of water.

Blended into fuel, ethanol burns more cleanly than pure gasoline, reducing fossil fuel dependence. It has powered vehicles for over a century due to its high octane rating when blended with petrol.

Comprising countless solutions, alcohol (particularly ethanol and isopropanol) dissolves substances from oils to pigments. It quickly evaporates, leaving surfaces clean. This makes it an extremely versatile solvent used across industries from manufacturing to medicine.

The unique chemical properties of the ethanol form of alcohol (ethanol is what we consume as 'drinking alcohol') have proven invaluable over centuries of human innovation. We have only begun to tap into alcohol's potential (e.g., its use as a biofuel) to advance progress.

Brilliant stuff! Incredibly useful.

The Pros: Alcohol the Beverage

In the interests of providing an objective discussion of the role of alcohol in society, it's important to also acknowledge the positive aspects of moderate alcohol consumption, especially in the context of cultural and social traditions.

Alcoholic beverages, such as wine, have played a vital role in cultural and social rituals for centuries, enriching ceremonies, celebrations and religious practices with their presence. Beyond tradition, alcohol can foster social bonding, often acting as a catalyst for camaraderie and communication in social settings. Sharing in these experiences often deepens connections, fostering meaningful relationships among individuals. And, when consumed in moderation, alcoholic beverages can offer personal enjoyment and relaxation, providing a moment of respite to unwind and savour moments of leisure. Some might suggest that this enhances the fabric of everyday life.

Alcoholic beverages, including wine, beer, gin, whisky and others, offer a dual benefit of culinary enjoyment and cultural significance. Paired with food, they elevate the dining experience for some by complementing a wide range of cuisines and dish types with their diverse flavours and sensory experiences. Moreover, wine in particular holds a rich historical and artistic significance and has been celebrated in art, literature and music throughout the ages. Often associated with creativity and cultural expression, it serves as both a muse for artists and a symbol of cultural heritage, at times enriching human experiences and fostering appreciation for the arts.

Some studies suggest that moderate alcohol consumption may offer certain health benefits, including cardiovascular benefits, improved heart health and a potential decrease in the risk of certain diseases (Chiva-Blanch & Badimon, 2019). While it pains us to include this statement, as we're highly sceptical that this is the case (when considered alongside healthy options that do not include alcohol, for instance), in the interests of objectivity it must be included!

Throughout history, the trade of alcoholic beverages has served as a vibrant collage of cultural exchange, melding together traditions, techniques and flavours from around the world. The legacy of this today manifests in regions celebrated for their wine-making or brewing traditions, drawing tourists to experience the rich local culture and invigorating economies. Furthermore, the production and distribution of alcoholic beverages forms a vital element in the framework of the global economy, nurturing agricultural sectors, sustaining manufacturing industries and infusing hospitality scenes with dynamic vitality. Thus, from its storied past of cultural exchange to its dynamic role in contemporary economies, alcohol continues to infuse life and flavour into communities worldwide.

The question remains: Should we really be ingesting something used to dissolve oil?

The Cons: Unmoderated Alcohol Intake Misuse

Collectively, most of us are familiar with the negative social and personal consequences associated with excessive alcohol consumption, often viewing them as afflictions that primarily affect others while maintaining a sense of distance from our own habits. To spell out the downsides of unmoderated alcohol consumption, many people would be aware of the following (in no particular order):

- **Addiction and dependence:** The addictive nature of alcohol means that prolonged and heavy consumption can result in both physical and psychological dependence, leading to conditions such as alcohol use disorder (AUD) or addiction.

- **Withdrawal symptoms:** When individuals who are dependent on alcohol suddenly stop their intake, they may experience withdrawal symptoms like anxiety, tremors, hallucinations and even seizures.

- **Impaired judgement and accidents:** Overindulgence in alcohol (through inhalation or drinking) can compromise cognitive functions and coordination skills. This raises the risk of accidents or injuries because of impaired decision-making capabilities – a situation that becomes particularly dangerous when activities like driving are involved.

- **Family and social issues:** Not only does excessive drinking strain relationships, causing family problems and social isolation, but it also leads to conflicts that can negatively affect an individual's personal life as well as their professional standing.

- **Mental health impact:** Alcohol misuse often correlates with increased instances of mental health disorders such as depression and anxiety – in addition, it has the potential to worsen pre-existing mental health conditions.

- **Violence and aggression:** A direct correlation exists between alcohol consumption levels and an increased likelihood of violent behaviour – this contributes not just to domestic violence but also to other aggressive acts such as assault.

- **Legal consequences:** Offences related to alcohol use, including DUIs (driving under the influence), public intoxication or disorderly conduct, could lead to legal repercussions ranging from fines or licence suspension all the way up to imprisonment.

- **Economic burden:** The societal costs associated with issues stemming from alcohol abuse – healthcare expenses, law enforcement requirements and lost productivity, to name a few – place a significant economic burden on both communities and governments.

- **Risk of overdose:** Extreme alcohol consumption can result in alcohol poisoning, which is potentially fatal. Symptoms may include confusion, vomiting, seizures, irregular breathing patterns or even loss of consciousness.

So, we may not personally be drinking to these levels. That's a relief! But wait – there's more.

The Cons: Lesser Known Health and Wellbeing Impacts

Cancer Risk

Alcohol consumption, particularly in excess, has long been recognised as a risk factor for various health issues, including liver diseases, cardiovascular problems and neurological impairment. We now know it is also a risk factor for certain cancers. Among the cancers associated with alcohol intake, breast cancer stands out as one of the most well-documented. Let's delve into the evidence linking ethanol, the type of alcohol found in alcoholic beverages, to breast cancer risk.

Facts

- **Classification by the International Agency for Research on Cancer (IARC):** The IARC, a part of the World Health Organization (WHO), classified alcoholic beverages as a Group 1 carcinogen in 1988. This classification signifies that there is sufficient evidence to conclude that alcohol consumption does cause cancer in humans.

- **Breast cancer risk:** Numerous studies have consistently shown a positive association between alcohol consumption and an increased risk of breast cancer. This risk appears to be dose-dependent, meaning that higher levels of alcohol intake are associated with a greater increase in breast cancer risk (McDonald et al., 2013).

- **Mechanisms of action:** The exact mechanisms by which alcohol increases breast cancer risk are not fully understood. However, alcohol may influence hormone levels, particularly estrogen, and may also exert direct toxic effects on cells.

- **Hormonal influence:** Alcohol consumption is known to elevate estrogen levels in the body, which have been linked to an increased risk of hormone receptor-positive breast cancers.

- **Other cancers:** Besides breast cancer, alcohol consumption has also been linked to an increased risk of other cancers, including those of the liver, colorectum, oesophagus and mouth.

Take Away

The link between alcohol consumption and breast cancer risk is well-established. It seems the overall risk to any individual may vary depending on factors such as the amount and frequency of alcohol consumed, genetic predisposition and other lifestyle factors. Of course, we generally understand that moderate alcohol consumption may carry a lower risk compared to heavy drinking. However, the evidence underscores the importance of being aware of these cold, hard facts when it comes to making decisions for our wellbeing.

Other Health and Wellbeing Risks

Despite the large part alcohol plays in the lives of many of us, the reality is that excessive alcohol intake can have detrimental effects on many and varied aspects of our general health. Understanding the breadth of these impacts is crucial for making informed decisions about our own alcohol consumption in order to safeguard our wellbeing.

Facts

- **Liver disease:** A study published in 2017 shows that excessive alcohol consumption is a leading cause of liver disease. This means that drinking too much alcohol can seriously harm your liver, an organ that plays a crucial role in digestion and detoxification. Conditions like fatty liver disease, alcoholic hepatitis and cirrhosis can result from alcohol-induced inflammation and damage to liver cells (Osna et al., 2017).

- **Heart disease:** Research published in *Alcohol Research: Current Reviews* indicates a strong link between heavy drinking and heart disease. Excessive alcohol intake can elevate blood pressure, disrupt heart rhythm and increase the risk of heart failure (Piano, 2017).

- **Obesity:** Studies suggest a correlation between alcohol consumption and obesity. Heavy drinkers are more likely to be obese due to the high calorie content of alcohol and its contribution to weight gain (Traversy & Chaput, 2018).

- **Brain health:** Alcohol doesn't just affect the liver, heart and body weight; it can also impact brain function. Chronic (long-term) heavy drinking can lead to cognitive impairment, memory loss and an increased risk of dementia. The study 'Alcohol Consumption and Cognitive Decline in Early Old Age' (Sabia et al., 2014) found that middle-aged men who drank more than 36 grams of alcohol per day (equivalent to two and a half standard drinks) experienced a faster cognitive decline over a 10-year period compared to light or moderate drinkers. This suggests that heavy drinking can speed up the ageing process of the brain. A study in 2001 found that heavy drinking could increase the risk of Alzheimer's disease, especially in people who have a genetic predisposition to the disease. This study suggests that alcohol may interact with the genes associated with Alzheimer's, increasing the risk of developing the disease (Tyas, 2001).

Take Away

From liver damage to heart disease, and from obesity to brain health and mental health issues, alcohol can have far-reaching consequences. It's essential to be mindful of alcohol intake and prioritise moderation to safeguard long-term health. Every decision regarding alcohol consumption plays a role in shaping our health outcomes, making informed choices crucial for a healthier lifestyle.

Damage to Teeth and Oral Health Risk

How many people have a detailed understanding of how alcohol can affect our teeth as well as our heads and livers? Here's a closer look at how alcohol consumption can impact our teeth and oral health.

Facts

- **Alcohol and tooth decay:** Studies have shown that alcohol consumption, especially of acidic beverages like wine, can contribute to dental erosion. The acidity in alcohol can wear away the protective enamel of our teeth, leading to sensitivity and cavities (Tezal et al., 2001).

- **Gum disease:** Alcohol can dry out the mouth, reducing saliva production, which plays a crucial role in washing away food particles and neutralising acids. This dryness can increase the risk of gum disease, a serious condition that can lead to tooth loss if left untreated.

- **Oral cancer:** As already indicated earlier on, heavy alcohol consumption has been linked to a higher risk of oral cancer. A study published in the *British Journal of Cancer* found that alcohol consumption is a significant risk factor for oral cancer. The researchers discovered that people who consume about four drinks per day have over twice the risk of developing oral cancer compared to non-drinkers. This means that moderating alcohol intake could potentially reduce the risk of oral cancer (Petti & Scully, 2005).

- **Bad breath:** Alcohol can cause bad breath by drying out the mouth, creating an environment where bacteria thrive.

- **Tooth staining:** Dark-coloured beverages like red wine and whisky can stain teeth, leading to discolouration.

- **Tooth sensitivity:** As alcohol erodes enamel, teeth can become more sensitive to hot and cold temperatures, making eating and drinking uncomfortable.

Take Away

While enjoying the occasional drink is unlikely to cause serious harm, regular heavy drinking, or sipping acidic beverages like wine often and over an extended period of time, can have significant negative effects on oral health. It's simply another fact to consider in the alcohol formula.

Effect on Sleep and Long-Term Brain Health Risk

Plenty of people will tell us that a 'nightcap' – having a drink or several in the evening –helps them drift off to sleep easily. However, research suggests otherwise.

There are multiple studies being done on sleep and it's an intriguing area of research. For so long we've taken sleep for granted – cutting back here and there to get in extra hours to plough through all the extra activities and tasks we have to get through in our modern lives. Lay on top of that our habits – perhaps including alcohol consumption in the evening – that actually undermine the quality of our sleep, and we're very likely doing ourselves some long-term damage.

Facts

- **Alcohol and rapid eye movement (REM) sleep:** A study found that alcohol suppresses REM sleep, the stage of sleep where dreams occur and memory consolidation takes place (Colrain et al., 2014). This could have serious implications for our memory and cognitive function in the long run. This information is backed up by Matthew Walker, a neuroscientist and sleep expert, in his book *Why We Sleep*, which reveals that alcohol disrupts REM sleep, which is crucial for memory consolidation and learning new things (Walker, 2017).

- **Alzheimer's disease risk:** A study found that during sleep, our brain clears out harmful toxins that can lead to Alzheimer's disease (Xie et al., 2013). Alcohol can disrupt this process, potentially increasing our risk of developing this much-feared disease. Again, Matthew Walker's work indicates that our brain cleanses itself of toxic metabolic by-products while we slumber, lack of which could lead to neurodegenerative diseases (Walker, 2017).

- **Alcohol and sleep apnoea:** A study found that alcohol relaxes the muscles in our throat, which can exacerbate sleep apnoea, a serious sleep disorder that causes one to stop breathing during sleep (Peppard et al., 2007). This can lead to a host of health problems, including heart disease and stroke.

Take Away

According to research, consumption of alcohol in a way that influences our sleep cycle, affects sleep negatively and leads to long-term poor and disrupted sleep has serious health implications. Some of these issues are the things many of us fear and pray we can avoid, such as looking old, losing our memory, having a stroke, getting Alzheimer's and reducing our lifespan, among a host of other things.

Foetal Alcohol Risk

Research is available that shows alcohol consumption during pregnancy can have detrimental effects on foetal health, with significant implications for both short-term and long-term outcomes. Several studies have highlighted the risks associated with prenatal alcohol exposure, and we'll outline a few of them below. While many people in the modern world will be extra careful of their health and diet during pregnancy, it seems likely that not everyone will know the importance of abstaining from alcohol during pregnancy to safeguard the wellbeing of the baby.

Facts

- **Preterm birth risk:** Research indicates that even moderate alcohol consumption during pregnancy can increase the risk of preterm birth, which may result in respiratory distress, feeding difficulties and heightened vulnerability to infections (Kesmodel et al., 2002).

- **Cognitive impacts:** Studies have shown that prenatal alcohol exposure, even at moderate levels, can adversely affect a child's cognitive development. Children exposed to alcohol in the womb may exhibit lower intelligence and academic achievement scores by the age of 10 (Sood et al., 2001).

- **Miscarriage, stillbirth and sudden infant death syndrome (SIDS):** Alcohol consumption during pregnancy has been linked to an elevated risk of miscarriage, stillbirth, preterm delivery and SIDS. These findings underscore the severe consequences of prenatal alcohol exposure and the imperative of abstaining from alcohol to safeguard foetal health (O'Leary et al., 2013).

Take Away

The evidence is now available: Prenatal alcohol exposure poses significant risks to foetal health and development. Alcohol is a teratogen, capable of causing birth defects and permanent cognitive impairments in the form of foetal alcohol syndrome (FAS). There is no safe amount of alcohol to drink during pregnancy, as any level of exposure can harm the developing baby. By abstaining from alcohol during pregnancy, women can ensure the best possible start in life for their children, protecting them from the irreversible consequences of prenatal alcohol exposure. If you're reading this book, I imagine you will agree that every decision matters when it comes to safeguarding the health and wellbeing of the next generation.

While moderate enjoyment with vigilance likely poses a low risk for some adults, the insights from emerging research warrant consideration of moderation – or even elimination from our diets. Alcohol's sociocultural halo often eclipses findings on its multifaceted biological impacts that we dismiss at our peril. Any substance with carcinogenic and addictive potential deserves a healthy respect... and possibly a wide berth.

Understanding the Big Picture

Why does this information help you? It's because as you go though life observing alcohol – the advertisements, friends consuming it, it featuring in movies and television shows, people talking about it (and talking about hangovers) – you can be mindful of its presence. Note it and contemplate what it is affecting – if it is. If you are thinking about having a drink or drinks, contemplate how you will feel afterwards.

I remember one of the most powerful things ever said to me at a time when I was in the thick of my struggle to drink–not drink. I was with a health coach discussing some self-care activities and she was telling me about drawing a beautiful deep bath, with essential oils and floating flowers and candles. I asked, 'I suppose it's not okay to have a glass of wine while having the bath?' and she told me, 'It's not about whether you should or shouldn't have wine – it's about asking yourself how you'll feel about it afterwards'. I knew how I'd feel about it, alright! And it wouldn't be good, because it wouldn't be just one!

From now, start to observe alcohol mindfully. Notice it and see how it exists around us.

Ideally, after absorbing the information in this chapter, you'll be forming a view of how much of your relationship with alcohol is filled with beneficial factors and how much is possibly harming you and all you hold dear. In the next chapter we'll have a look at why people develop issues with alcohol.

Chapter 2:

Why Do People Develop Issues With Alcohol?

In this chapter, we delve into the intricate web of factors that contribute to the development of unhealthy relationships with alcohol. While the journey that led us to this point, where alcohol holds sway over our lives, might have been confounding and frustrating, understanding its underlying dynamics is the first step towards empowerment and liberation. By unravelling these complexities, we gain the insights and tools necessary to reclaim control and break free from alcohol's grasp.

Problematic alcohol use is a multifaceted condition, shaped by a myriad of influences spanning biology, environment and psychology. Untangling the various strands requires a nuanced approach, one that acknowledges both the external and internal forces at play.

In the following pages, we'll navigate through the maze of environmental, social and cultural factors (which we'll refer to as external) and then the genetic, biological, psychological and personality factors (which we'll refer to as internal) that intertwine to mould individuals' relationships with alcohol. By shedding light on these external and internal influences, we aim to provide insight, clarity and, ultimately, a pathway towards breaking free from this damaging relationship and enabling greater well-being.

So, let's continue with this journey of becoming better informed of the facts, developing a greater understanding of the factors at play and allowing compassion for ourselves and this predicament we find ourselves in, as well as growth towards the future we want to have. Together, we'll help equip you with the knowledge and determination to pave a way towards a healthier, more fulfilling life – where you are in control of your wellbeing.

External Factors Influencing Unhealthy Relationships With Alcohol

While it's challenging to neatly separate environmental, social, and cultural factors, we'll strive to provide some clarity, acknowledging the overlap and interconnection among these terms. Our aim is to navigate through these complexities logically, offering a structured exploration for the sake of clarity.

Sensory Influences: Navigating Messages About Alcohol Consumption in Our Environment

Our modern, Western environment seems almost intentionally designed to foster alcohol dependence.

Accessibility

First, the sheer omnipresence of alcohol constantly creates a thirst for it. It's prominently displayed in or near grocery aisles, at petrol stations, at sporting events, on bus shelters and even on the buses themselves. There are even drive-through liquor stores! And neighbourhood bars, taverns, pubs and similar 'watering holes' dot street corners, wooing after-work crowds. With such incredibly easy accessibility, no wonder many people grab a six-pack with the same casualness as the household staples of bread and milk. Happy hours serve as enticing opportunities, offering discounted drinks as rewards for those seeking an earlier than usual initiation of their daily drinking ritual. Over time, cues for drinking easily become embedded into daily routine.

In the Home

At home, family habits pass alcohol appetites through generations, including around holidays and special events. Seeing mothers unwinding with wine daily or dads eagerly awaiting a 'cold one' after work firmly imprints the notion that drinking accompanies adulthood. Children observe coping mechanisms based on ever-flowing refills when stresses and pressures get intense. These dynamics sear into memories, laying neural pathways in the brain for hereditary overuse despite one's best intentions.

Peer Pressure and Influence

Later, as we make new connections, our peers may encourage us to join in drinking games or 'shots' as part of bonding rituals, often equating moderation with dullness. Eager to break away from our high school personas, many of us may find ourselves overindulging at social gatherings, fearing exclusion if we don't partake and influenced by pervasive messages that link drinking with attractiveness and popularity on college campuses and in workplaces. Even as we transition into our professional lives, the pressure to unwind with alcohol after a stressful day remains prevalent, with colleagues often normalising daily drinks as a way to cope with the pressures of the job – particularly in environments where performance demands are high and job security feels uncertain.

Advertising and Promotion

Throughout life's journey, the media aggressively reinforces drinking ideals in flashy posters, print media, billboards and TV. From music stars downing champagne in videos to big game commercials selling beer as essential for true fandom, these perpetual messages embed drinking as integral for peak experiences. Even product placement in films makes cocktails and other enticing concoctions ever-present temptations. If you've ever been tempted by the '2 for 1' deal, you'll know what I mean. Free tasting at airport lounges? Why not! Purchased a new pair of shoes? What are the chances there'll be a $100 voucher for the latest greatest wine club included in the packaging? Too bad if you're trying to not think about drinking.

Misinformation in the General Media

Misinformation about alcohol, particularly the notion of its health benefits, continues to circulate in the media, despite being debunked by more recent research. A prime example of this is the commonly quoted health claims about red wine being beneficial due to the presence of resveratrol, a compound with potential anti-inflammatory and antioxidant properties. However, these claims are often based on selective reporting of findings from studies that have since been called into question.

A study published in the *Journal of Studies on Alcohol and Drugs*, which analysed 87 previous studies on alcohol consumption and mortality, found that moderate drinkers might not have the mortality advantage once thought. The researchers discovered that earlier studies may have compared moderate drinkers (those who consume up to two drinks per day) to a group that included individuals who had cut down or stopped drinking due to poor health, potentially skewing the results and making moderate drinking seem healthier than it actually is (Stockwell et al., 2016).

Furthermore, a study titled 'Alcohol and Mortality: A Cohort Study' found that while moderate alcohol consumption was associated with a lower risk of mortality, the benefits were outweighed by the risks, which included liver disease, cancer and accidents (Kono et al., 1986). This means that while a glass of wine might not be harmful, it's not necessarily beneficial either.

It's crucial to be critical of claims about the health benefits of alcohol and to rely on updated, evidence-based information regarding its effects on health. The media's selective reporting of findings can lead to the perpetuation of misinformation, which can have serious consequences for public health. It is essential to consider the full body of research and to approach claims about the health benefits of alcohol with a critical eye.

With such overbearing sensory bombardment, the cultural reflex after constant exposure becomes 'I just need a drink' or 'It's normal to drink'. But despite promises of relaxation, happiness and even relief from life's stresses from all those ads, alcohol dependence often delivers the opposite long-term. Yet the environmental nudges towards unhealthy use remain so relentless that conscious effort is essential to recognise and resist the manipulation. We must see through the illusions... easier said than done within society's breathless intoxication! But with self-reflection, critical thinking and compassion for ourselves and others, we can find the inner clarity needed to break free.

Conditioning Influences: Understanding Social and Cultural Messages About Alcohol

The general environment in certain countries can angle people towards unhealthy drinking. Layered on top of that, social pressures and cultural messages also potently sway our decisions, often without us realising it. Our primitive brain's tribal wiring to belong makes overriding cultural norms an exhausting, seemingly unsurmountable battle

Rituals

Across life's stages, rituals reinforce alcohol as indispensable for connecting through 'Cheers', 'Salute', 'Salud', 'Prost' or 'Yamas'. As teens, those abstaining from parties feel branded as outsiders. In adulthood, wine-free dinner guests confront awkward questions about why they aren't imbibing like everyone else. The default expectation becomes constant-flow refills... anything else seems to require justification. Perhaps you're aware that the default silver service table setting includes wine glasses, which are taken away if you do not drink – rather than the appropriate glasses being added if you do drink. Have you ever tried to explain that you'd like to drink your water from the pretty wine glass while dining, and not the boring water glass? It's just too confusing and simply not the 'done thing'. Trying to extract oneself from rituals that are so deeply engrained is not easy!

Gifts and Thanks

What to give for a gift? Wine, sparkling or still. Spirits, proof, aged, oaked and blended. There is a bottle of alcohol to suit all occasions! Furthermore, there are bottle-shaped gift bags to deliver them in – no need for wrapping! Problem easily solved! Even professionals gift wine to clients, assuming universal appeal. Many people, even those who have struggled with addiction in the past, reluctantly accept offers of alcohol for fear of offending others. How easily people get entangled by innocuous intentions.

Rewards and Benefits

Additionally, cruise lines and resorts frame alcohol as essential for vacation fun, bundling 'value-added' drink packages. Does that mean I get cold-pressed juices as a substitute offer for my cruise bonus if I do not partake in alcohol? Probably not… Sheesh, it's not easy taking the healthy option, is it?

Culture of Ego-Related Drinking

In bars, peer pressure towards 'shots' brands holdouts as party poopers. Machismo cultures particularly vaunt drinking prowess as proof of manliness, shaming abstinence. Across so many social spheres, conformity burnout overwhelms individual care and effort.

Tragically, the young suffer some of the worst effects of this culture given their developmental vulnerability. Teen exposure during critical neurogenesis can forever blunt cognitive potential. Yet high school drinking gets dismissed as 'just part of growing up' despite its life-altering risks. Parents cave to the tide of normalisation instead of succumbing to their intuitive nurturing instinct and acting to protect maturing minds.

Social coercion adds intense friction against self-care, allowing alcoholism's popularity to keep spreading unconsciously through populations over generations. Only by recognising conformity's manipulative ways can people consciously reclaim their control. We must offer patient space for each individual's choices without pressures either way, for preservation of health and dignity necessitates freedom from the herd's hurried pace towards destruction. The more of us who awaken to social programming, the more newcomers can smoothly walk their own path.

Internal Factors Influencing Unhealthy Relationships With Alcohol

A little investigation uncovers evidence that certain genetic, biological, psychological and personality factors render some people more vulnerable to alcohol dependence than others. Knowing a little about these factors gives us incredibly powerful information to work with.

Genetics

Research indicates that genetics helps determine our neurochemistry's interaction with alcohol. A study conducted by the National Institute on Alcohol Abuse and Alcoholism found that genetics accounts for about half of the risk of alcoholism (Schuckit, 2009). The researchers uncovered that certain genes increase a person's risk, while others may decrease that risk, directly influencing a person's susceptibility to alcoholism. This means that if a person has a family history of alcoholism, they could be more likely to develop the same problem. However, it's not a guarantee, as environmental factors also play a significant role. There is also a suggestion that just because a person's parents or grandparents were alcoholics, it doesn't necessarily mean they will be too. The genetic predisposition to alcoholism can skip generations, showing up in later generations due to the combination of genetic and environmental factors.

So, if – like I did, before I increased my knowledge about this – you find it a challenge to keep away from drinking alcohol or moderate your intake, it simply means that your genetic makeup may mean you are more susceptible to the rewarding effects of alcohol, making it harder for you to resist its allure. It is not a moral failing!

Or, if you've ever found yourself fretfully wondering why your friend seems to be oblivious to the fact that their glass of sparkling wine has lasted at least an hour, then the genetic factor may be one of the reasons you're struggling to hold back from your third or fourth in the same time frame – and thinking about it every second of that hour. Alternatively, it could be partly due to the fact that you're used to being around your usual family environment, where a bottle of sparkling wine is downed between two ladies in the space of an hour. Noting these experiences from the past and becoming observant about the presence of and influence of alcohol all around you – as well as how you feel about it when you interact with it (and after you've interacted with it) – is going to be a powerful tool for you to take with you from this point forward.

Interestingly, studies show certain ethnicities possess lower alcohol tolerance due to differing metabolisation, which causes toxicity symptoms rather than euphoria. This predisposition arises from a reduced ability to metabolise alcohol effectively due to certain genetic variants of the enzymes alcohol dehydrogenase (ADH) and aldehyde dehydrogenase (ALDH). Higuchi et al. (1996) conducted a study that revealed individuals possessing the *ALDH2*2* variant were less likely to engage in heavy drinking due to the unpleasant symptoms they experienced, such as facial flushing and nausea. These symptoms result from the accumulation of acetaldehyde – a toxic by-product of alcohol metabolism – in the bloodstream. The prevalence of this type of genetic variant among Native American and Australian Aboriginal populations as well as East Asian populations suggests a genetic predisposition towards alcohol intolerance in these individuals.

Biology

There is no need for concern about willpower or moral strength – what we're clarifying here involves the intricate dance of chemicals in our brains and how they interact with substances like alcohol. For example, the research study 'Alcohol and the Brain: Neuronal Molecular Targets,

Synapses, and Circuits' delved into the nitty-gritty of how alcohol affects neurotransmitters in the brain, which are responsible for transmitting signals that influence our mood and behaviour (Abrahao et al., 2017). You probably won't be surprised to know that alcohol can increase the release of dopamine, a neurotransmitter associated with pleasure and reward, which can make drinking feel good. Logically, this action and reaction can potentially lead to addiction in some people. There is another study, 'The Role of GABA in the Pathophysiology and Treatment of Anxiety Disorders', which explored the role of GABA, a neurotransmitter that inhibits brain activity and promotes relaxation. The findings? Alcohol enhances the effects of GABA, leading to feelings of calm and relaxation (Nemeroff, 2003). So, over time, the brain may become reliant on alcohol to stimulate GABA production, leading to addiction. Again, these are just a few of the many facts now known about ethyl alcohol and the human brain.

I don't know about you, but I find comfort in this knowledge. It's enlightening and empowering. It explains things I previously didn't understand and makes me feel better about myself and my previous struggles – a tremendous boost for self-compassion and self-esteem. You may not feel the same – yet – but let's persevere.

Psychological Factors

The research shows that psychological factors play a crucial role in predisposing individuals to alcoholism, with underlying mental health conditions often serving as significant contributors. Studies have shed light on the intricate relationship between psychological disorders and alcohol use disorders (Palzes et al., 2020). When we're looking to understand the pathway we've come down to end up with a dependence on alcohol that we didn't expect, unveiling these compelling insights is incredibly helpful.

Anxiety

For instance, a study by Kushner et al. (2005) demonstrated that individuals with anxiety disorders are more likely to develop alcohol dependence. The researchers suggested that individuals may use alcohol as a form of self-medication to alleviate anxiety symptoms, ultimately leading to addiction. This finding underscores the importance of treating anxiety disorders to mitigate the risk of alcoholism. When, in subsequent chapters, we start talking about quitting drinking, this explains why we need to come up with a plan that covers all of our needs – a holistic approach. It's a bit like going on a vegan diet – you can't just cut out meat and keep eating the other foods you've always eaten! That leaves certain needs of the person completely unmet.

Childhood Experiences

Similarly, research has found a strong correlation between childhood trauma and the development of alcohol dependence later in life (Brady & Back, 2012). This study emphasised that traumatic experiences in childhood significantly increase the risk of alcoholism in adulthood, highlighting the importance of early intervention and support for children who have experienced trauma to potentially prevent future alcohol addiction.

Big T or little t

The world of psychology and mental health is a maze of terms and concepts, each with its own nuances and implications. One such distinction that has been gaining attention in recent years is the differentiation between 'childhood trauma with a capital T' and 'childhood trauma with a lower case t' (Burri et al., 2013; Afifi et al., 2008).

This distinction, while seemingly minor, can have profound implications for understanding, diagnosing and treating individuals who have experienced traumatic events in their early years.

'Childhood trauma with a capital T' often refers to severe, life-threatening or catastrophic events that are widely recognised as traumatic, such as physical or sexual abuse, neglect, natural disasters or witnessing violence. These experiences are typically more overt and extreme in nature, leading to significant psychological distress and long-term consequences for the individual's mental and emotional wellbeing.

On the other hand, 'childhood trauma with a lower case t' may encompass a broader range of adverse experiences and stressors that can also have a significant impact on a child's development and mental health, but may not meet the criteria for severe or overt trauma. This could include experiences such as parental divorce, chronic illness, bullying, emotional neglect or other forms of family dysfunction. While these experiences may be less extreme or overt, they can still have profound effects on a child's psychological and emotional development, potentially leading to issues such as anxiety, depression or difficulties in forming healthy relationships later in life.

Both types of childhood trauma, whether with a capital T or a lower case t, can have lasting effects on individuals and may contribute to an increased risk of mental health problems, including substance abuse and addiction, later in life. It's important for individuals who have experienced any form of childhood trauma to seek support and appropriate treatment to address the impact of these experiences on their wellbeing.

Depression

Moreover, a study revealed that individuals with psychiatric disorders, particularly mood disorders like depression and bipolar disorder, are at heightened risk of developing alcohol use disorders (Palzes et al., 2020). This underscores the notion that mental health conditions may predispose individuals to alcoholism, highlighting the importance of addressing mental health issues in alcohol addiction treatment.

Overall, these studies illuminate the intricate interplay between psychological factors and alcohol addiction, emphasising the importance of addressing underlying mental health conditions in addiction prevention and treatment.

A particular point I'd like to highlight is the tendency some of us have to downplay factors that lead to distress – for which some of us may unknowingly choose to 'self-medicate' with alcohol. We know we are 'lucky' because we have a roof over our heads, clothes to wear, food to eat and, to a large extent, choices in life. We have not had capital T childhood trauma and, although we may be a bit anxious and stressed, we 'don't have anything to complain about'. Thus, we shouldn't be self-medicating and shouldn't get addicted. Are you with me? In the interests of self-compassion and taking care of the whole person, do take note of the very real potential of 'little t' childhood trauma to leave some of us a little fragile and a little ill-equipped to overcome challenges, achieve our goals and foster resilience. We certainly don't want to 'wallow in self-pity' or 'play the victim role' – because our wellbeing and healing starts with us! But when we start to address a plan for quitting drinking and taking care of the whole person, personal development and taking steps to optimise our mental health must be a part of that plan, whether we seek out a coach, therapist or other guide or go it alone with appropriate resources. We'll get onto this in Chapter 5.

Stress and Coping Mechanisms

No surprises here – alcohol is often used as a coping mechanism in the absence of knowledge of a healthier way. High levels of everyday stress and an inability to cope with life's challenges just seem to drive many of us to seek solace in alcohol as a distraction from the feelings we can't seem to cope with. Stress, loneliness, sadness, anger, frustration, anxiety and other negative emotions need to be dealt with. And if we don't have a healthy coping mechanism we know how to use, turning to alcohol instead can lead to a cycle of dependence and perhaps, eventually, addiction.

We'd like to point out that not having healthy coping mechanisms isn't generally any fault of our own – after all, we're not taught 'emotions management' in school! Healthy emotional coping mechanisms are crucial and in later chapters we will discuss a variety of these, such as exercise, mindfulness, meditation, hobbies and more. The good news is, sometimes the most powerful methods are also the most readily available, and often the most affordable.

To provide an example of how this comes into play, one study focused on the *GABRA2* gene, which affects the brain's GABA system, which helps regulate our response to stress and anxiety. The researchers found that variations in this gene are associated with a higher risk of alcohol dependence (Edenberg, 2013). This suggests that people with these variations might turn to alcohol as a way to cope with stress and anxiety, increasing their risk of addiction.

Personality Traits

Personality traits appear to play a significant role in shaping individuals' relationship with alcohol, as evidenced by numerous scientific studies.

A meta-analysis (a research method used to combine and analyse the results of multiple independent studies on a particular topic) revealed a compelling correlation between impulsivity and alcohol consumption (Shin et al., 2012). The study concluded that individuals with higher levels of impulsivity are more prone to heavy drinking and developing alcohol-related problems, suggesting that managing impulsivity could be crucial in preventing alcohol addiction.

Similarly, another study uncovered that sensation-seeking individuals are more likely to consume alcohol and encounter alcohol-related issues (Scott & Corbin, 2014). This finding implies that interventions targeting sensation-seeking behaviours could prove beneficial in mitigating alcohol addiction risks.

Furthermore, a study identified four distinct personality profiles based on major traits. Of these profiles, the one characterised by high neuroticism (reflecting a greater tendency to experience heightened emotional reactivity and vulnerability to stress) and low conscientiousness (reflecting fewer traits associated with organisation, responsibility and self-discipline) exhibited the highest level of alcohol consumption, indicating that certain personality profiles may be more susceptible to alcohol addiction (Jemberie et al., 2020).

Delving deeper into the subject, it's intriguing to note that personality traits tend to remain stable throughout adulthood. This means that individuals who display impulsivity or sensation-seeking tendencies in their youth are likely to continue exhibiting these traits into adulthood, potentially influencing their susceptibility to alcohol addiction.

Lack of Support Systems

Research has shown that people with limited social support systems, isolation and a lack of healthy coping mechanisms are more likely to succumb to alcohol dependence. Let's study the science behind this.

One study found that people with stronger social support networks were more likely to maintain a new path without alcohol (Lookatch et al., 2019). The researchers found that those with a strong network of friends and family who supported their recovery were less likely to relapse into alcohol use. So, this suggests that having a strong support system can be a protective factor against alcohol dependence.

Further supporting this evidence is a study that shows a strong correlation between social isolation and alcohol use. The researchers found that people who felt isolated were more likely to use alcohol as a coping mechanism (Wakabayashi et al., 2022). It won't be surprising to you that this suggests feelings of loneliness and isolation can contribute to alcohol dependence.

Thankfully, having support systems doesn't just mean having friends and family around. It can also come from support groups, therapists, coaches and other sources of emotional support – social support can come in many forms.

Neural Pathways and Habits

As an avid researcher, I've become fascinated by the world of neural pathways and habits, particularly focusing on how the ritual of, say, having a drink at a certain time of day can become a habit that further strengthens the relationship with alcohol.

Research has found that habitual behaviours are driven by neural pathways in the brain. These pathways become stronger each time the behaviour is repeated, making the habit harder to break (Smith & Laiks, 2018).

So, not only do we have our brain chemistry telling us it's time for a drink in the afternoon, our neural pathways have become accustomed to the ritual as well! Sure as the dog is drooling at the back door for her dinner bowl to be filled, our need for that ritual of the evening drink kicks in. If the chemical addiction is not difficult enough to deal with, we have this additional challenge to work on! But the good news is, the same process can be used to form healthier habits. By consistently repeating a healthier behaviour at the same time each day, we can create new neural pathways that eventually become stronger than the old ones.

A study found that people who used a technique called 'implementation intentions' were more successful at breaking habits (Adriaanse et al., 2011). This involves planning ahead and deciding exactly what you will do in a situation where you're tempted to fall back into your old habit. For example, if your old habit was having a drink at 5 p.m., you might decide to go for a walk or drink a glass of water at that time instead. I admit, I do find this laughable as a stand-alone suggestion. Anyone who suggests to us, when we have not yet broken free of the claws of alcohol, to go for a walk instead, or have a glass of water instead, simply have no comprehension of what it's like, do they? A well-meaning family doctor I broached about the subject of my distress over not being able to moderate my alcohol intake, despite my best efforts, suggested the 'go for a walk' solution. I don't think I have ever felt so misunderstood and so alone as I did at that point. But stick with me, because I can tell you that now I look forward to my sparkling water with a big squeeze of lemon or lime juice at the end of the day, and I do not miss the wine. It's a bit of a process, but it's possible. And, looking back, I have far more knowledge, tools and support resources than I had back then, and they're all here in this book to make it a whole lot easier for you!

You may already have heard these figures, but a study titled 'Making Health Habitual: The Psychology of 'Habit-Formation' and General Practice' published in the *British Journal of General Practice* found that it takes an average of 66 days to form a new habit (Gardner et al., 2012). So, it's going to feel a little uncomfortable to make this change. A habit can be like a superhighway in our brain! It takes a bit of planning and resolve to put a detour sign in place and make a new habit stick by consistently practising it – but, eventually, a new habit can become as automatic and deeply entrenched as your old one.

Whatever the Reasons, the Result and the Way Forward Are the Same

Alcohol dependence is a complex issue involving a combination of genetic, environmental and psychological factors. And each of these factors can be seemingly as strong and difficult to overcome as the next. What's useful to know is that a dependence on alcohol often co-occurs with emotional and mental health issues. We don't feel great, we don't have a way to feel better and deal with the underlying issue – which quite often we don't even realise *is* an underlying issue – and alcohol can be a welcome distraction, allowing us a little respite from our uncomfortable emotions for a time. It seems like alcohol can temporarily reduce the symptoms of stress, anxiety or depression, but it is known that in the long term, alcohol use can actually worsen these conditions. It may not surprise you to know that other distractions – excessive shopping, overeating, gaming, gambling and TV watching, to name a few – can also serve the same purpose and become similarly problematic. And similarly, with the right knowledge, a sound, holistic plan, the right support and, sometimes, additional treatment, liberation from a dependence on alcohol is possible. Many people successfully overcome alcohol dependence and continue on with healthy, fulfilling lives.

We've now covered a lot of facts about what alcohol is, where it came from, the pros and cons and why some people become addicted to it and some do not. In the next chapter, we'll take a closer look at our motivations for quitting drinking and the reasons behind our decision to remove alcohol from our lives. This introspective journey will help us gain clarity and strengthen our resolve as we move forward on this transformative path.

Following that, we'll explore the various options available for quitting drinking, including strategies for managing any cravings and withdrawal symptoms that may arise after eliminating alcohol from our system. We'll also discuss effective ways to cope with the challenges of maintaining sobriety in the long run, ensuring that our commitment to a healthier, alcohol-free lifestyle remains strong and unwavering.

Chapter 3:

Your 'Why' for Quitting Drinking

When it comes to re-evaluating our drinking habits (or any habits, in fact), it's crucial to first get clear on the underlying reasons driving the need for change. In other words, what experiences, goals or incentives are stirring self-inquiry about your relationship with alcohol? Pinpointing your motivation will provide the clarity and conviction that are essential to stay the course when the path gets challenging.

In this chapter, we'll reflect deeply on four key areas to help unearth your personal 'why' for exploring the option of quitting drinking:

- **Health and longevity:** Is alcohol conflicting with your aim of extending your active, vibrant years?

- **Quality of life:** Might alcohol drain your everyday energy and vibrancy rather than enhancing it? We'll delve into the effects of alcohol on daily life.

- **Being a positive role model:** If you mentor young people, you likely worry about indirectly shaping their assumptions. We'll confront the tough realities all caregivers face.

- **Nurturing relationships:** It's common for problem drinking to quietly strain close connections. We'll investigate how it obstructs human connection and intimacy.

Of course, your 'why' around changing your habits could blend several of these motivations or include other incentives not listed. The goal of this chapter is simply to draw on the facts covered in Chapters 1 and 2 to spark insightful self-inquiry that reveals your unique and distinctive reasons, wherever that may lead. Illuminating why this exploration is meaningful and important to you will help you stay committed and motivated when obstacles arise.

Do You Want to Live Longer?

An important question to ask ourselves is, 'Do I want to live a long, healthy life, without dying prematurely?'

As we saw in Chapter 1, the emerging research reveals that consistent heavy drinking can significantly increase risks of serious health issues, potentially shortening one's lifespan. From heightened cancer vulnerability to earlier onset of cognitive decline, the compound impacts of long-term overconsumption should give anyone pause.

While moderate alcohol intake may fall within acceptable boundaries for some adults, it's wise to examine whether your personal consumption habits are pushing the limits of what's considered relatively low risk. For example, carefully consider the research that links even low-level daily drinking to an increased risk of certain cancers – including breast, colon, oesophageal and liver cancer. Ideally, don't turn a blind eye to the fact that alcohol has been clearly identified as a Group 1 carcinogen – the highest risk category.

Additionally concerning is the clear evidence of alcohol's detrimental impact on sleep quality. Keep in mind that while nightcaps can hasten initial snoozing, studies reveal that alcohol subsequently suppresses REM and slow-wave sleep, which is critical for cognition, metabolism and immunity (Colrain et al., 2014). Even marginal sleep disruption cumulatively increases vulnerability over decades. Poor sleep also heightens the risk of dementia and Alzheimer's disease onset later in life. We barely scraped the surface of the evidence that exists around this topic.

So, if living actively into your 80s, 90s and beyond appeals to you, limiting alcohol intake – or quitting entirely – may significantly stack the odds in your favour. In your decision as to the place alcohol has (or does not have) in your life, keep foremost to mind that the emerging data confirms that the less you drink, the better it is for longevity, cancer prevention and cognitive health.

Do You Want to Live a Healthier Existence?

There's a major difference between purely extending life span versus actually enhancing quality of life. It's the distinction between truly living vibrantly and merely surviving, marked by frequent medical appointments, reliance on medication and a persisting list of ailments to manage. The goal isn't simply surviving more years, but thriving with energy and vigour for as long as possible. I don't know about you, but I've never claimed to be 'here for a good time, not a long time' – I'm aiming for a good time *and* a long time!

So, consider – would curbing or quitting drinking allow you to more fully embrace daily wellness and vibrancy? Are you currently at a healthy, stable weight – or do excess alcohol calories tip the scales? Be honest about whether drinking habits displace nutritious food in your diet. And while the occasional indulgence adds joy, take stock if hangovers regularly steal productivity and happy moods.

Also, when having annual health assessments and screening blood tests with your general practitioner – always a good idea, especially as we advance in age – examine the results. Are biomarkers like liver enzymes, blood glucose and cholesterol at optimal levels? Or could alcohol be silently encroaching on your internal systems? Don't ignore early warnings just because outward symptoms aren't yet apparent.

And scrutinise your sleep honestly – with alcohol affecting life-affirming sleep foundations, are you waking rested, renewed and ready to embrace each day with gusto? Or do you slog through mornings foggy and depleted from partial sleep deprivation? Curbing drinking may feel difficult initially, but the long-term energy dividend is immense.

The goal is to not just tally days on a calendar, but to actually fill those days with peak experiences and effervescence. If alcohol shadows that aim, reassess its role – more years of muddling through life lethargically short-changes your potential. Prioritise daily wellbeing, adaptability and lightness of being.

Some other questions to ask yourself might be along the lines of: Am I reaching my career potential? Is my business success all it could be? Am I becoming a better version of myself each year?

What else would you add?

Do You Want to Set a Good Example for Those Around You Whom You Influence?

If you have children or mentor young people, it's natural to worry about indirectly influencing their future relationship with alcohol. Studies confirm that there is a cause for concern.

One such study found a strong correlation between the age at which a person first consumes alcohol and their likelihood of developing alcohol use disorder (AUD) later in life (Soundararajan et al., 2017). The researchers discovered that individuals who had their first drink at age 15 were four times more likely to develop AUD than those who waited until they were 21.

I recall with wry clarity the guilt I sometimes felt when neighbourhood kids caught me pouring an afternoon wine as I cooked dinner. While moderate drinking didn't yet feel problematic personally, I agonised over normalising daily consumption to impressionable young minds.

Our culture often overlooks how parents' casual drinking subtly shapes assumptions in children that drinking alcohol signifies relaxing and rewarding yourself. My own sons copied my wine-while-cooking habit with sparkling juice as tiny tots, innocent to the implications. Yet such play acting speaks volumes.

And even without overt mimicking, kids absorb behavioural modelling from caregivers around substance use far more than we realise. The data reveals that if a close relative struggles with alcohol, a child's statistical odds of developing those patterns heighten significantly.

So if you have any inkling that your drinking conflicts with setting a healthy example, listen to that inner voice. Protecting young people from early alcohol exposure gives them their best shot at avoiding hazardous habits down the road. Your conscientiousness today could spare loved ones suffering tomorrow.

The guilt I occasionally felt when kids caught me carelessly drinking reinforced that my evolving relationship with alcohol required re-evaluation. None of us wants generations copying behaviours that dimmed our own light. Make choices aligned with your highest aspirations for their welfare.

Do You Want to Have a Better Relationship With a Loved One... or Ones?

It's common for unhealthy drinking patterns to subtly strain close relationships – even without us realising the impacts in the moment. Reflect on whether alcohol causes you to miss out on meaningful time with loved ones.

For instance, do you ever catch yourself choosing to numb out on the couch with wine rather than actively engaging with family on weekends? I distinctly remember dozing off early on Friday after relaxing with a couple of wines while my kids were still up playing – precious hours I can never get back.

Or have friends and partners ever commented on your drinking interfering with intimacy or reliability? Consider if alcohol-influenced behaviours create emotional distance without you even noticing it at first.

Also scrutinise if drinking rituals restrict your schedule's flexibility overall. When the 5 o'clock glass of wine becomes non-negotiable, it dictates which activities make the cut. Hobbies, community events or travel ambitions may inadvertently get sidelined.

I vividly recall a holiday experience, sitting at a beachside location eating fish and chips for dinner with our sons and playing in the water park at a time of day when – prior to our decision to exclude drinking from our lives – it would have been 'drinkies time' and we would never have gone out. The feeling of fulfilment and liberation was euphoric.

And while drinking is often positioned as fun bonding among friends, pay attention if it begins to replace deeper relating. Foregoing vulnerable sharing or thoughtful conversations in favour of booze-fuelled banter risks real connection.

If your drinking feels misaligned with showing up fully available – emotionally and physically – for those who matter most, use that as inspiration to reassess its role in your life. Strengthening relationships through rediscovered presence ultimately proves far more rewarding than any drink.

The friends and family who offer unconditional love deserve your best self. Make space for joyful clarity and attunement the way only sobriety allows. Prioritise ever-evolving connection and intimacy on this wondrous – and one-off opportunity – journey of life together.

Defining Your 'Why'

While we're listing 'four possible whys', in reality, your 'why' may be a combination of two or more of these, or all of them – or something else entirely. The important point is to contemplate why you're exploring this topic. What is your longer-term vision for yourself? What's your 'why'?

Ultimately, only you can define the incentives that are most stirring and compelling for your life. So, we encourage deep introspection around your unique relationship with alcohol as it relates to your core values and future vision.

What daily existence do you envisage for the next phase of your life? How might shifting drinking patterns help manifest that goal? Whether they're centred on vitality, relationships, purpose or something else entirely, let your highest aspirations be the compass guiding your decisions.

Get quiet with yourself and listen to your inner wisdom. It may reveal nuances around your needs and trajectory that are not yet consciously apparent. Therein lies the beauty of self-inquiry – illuminating that which supports your continued expansion into the person you wish to become.

Trust that if reflecting on alcohol consumption patterns feels resonant, there is powerful insight awaiting discovery. Be gentle with yourself in this process – there are no rights or wrongs as you discern your distinctive 'why'. Wherever clarity takes you, embrace it as progress lighting your next steps from within.

Chapter 4:

Breaking Free From Alcohol—A Practical Look at Ways to Stop Drinking

For millions worldwide, the quest to quit drinking alcohol represents a transformative path from dependence or addiction to freedom, liberation, sobriety, healing and renewed purpose. It is a deeply personal journey that challenges individuals to confront not only their reliance on alcohol but also the underlying emotional, social and psychological factors that are contributing to it.

In this chapter, we will explore a diverse range of approaches to quitting drinking and examine the potential benefits and drawbacks of each. From the long-standing tradition of Alcoholics Anonymous (AA) to the so-called 'cold turkey' method, medication-assisted treatments, nutritional therapies and holistic lifestyle changes, there is no one-size-fits-all solution. Each approach offers unique perspectives, strategies and support systems that cater to the varied needs and preferences of those seeking to overcome alcohol dependence.

As we look into these options, we will provide insights into the fundamental beliefs, processes and practices that underpin each approach. We will also explore the scientific evidence and real-world implications of these methods and take a look at some personal experiences, offering a nuanced understanding of their effectiveness and limitations.

By examining the pros and cons of each approach, we aim to empower individuals with the additional knowledge and understanding necessary to make informed decisions about their path to a healthier future and the person they always imagined themselves to be — free from a dependence on alcohol.

Option 1: Alcoholics Anonymous

AA is a globally renowned mutual aid fellowship that provides support and guidance to individuals struggling with alcohol addiction. It was founded in 1935 by Bill Wilson, commonly known as Bill W., a former stockbroker whose own journey with alcoholism and eventual spiritual awakening became foundational to the programme, and Dr Bob Smith, a surgeon who, like Bill, achieved recovery from alcoholism and joined forces with him to establish AA. AA originated in Akron, Ohio, with the aim of offering a solution to alcoholism through a 12-step programme.

The core philosophy of AA revolves around mutual support and empathy among its members, who refer to themselves as 'alcoholics' or 'recovering alcoholics'. The programme emphasises the importance of admitting powerlessness over alcohol, surrendering to a higher power (often referred to as God, although the concept is interpreted in various ways) and taking personal inventory to address character defects. Central to AA's approach is the belief in abstinence from alcohol as the foundation for recovery.

AA operates through a decentralised structure, with over 115,000 autonomous support groups worldwide. These groups, attended by over two million members, meet regularly in diverse settings like churches, community centres or online platforms. Led by volunteers who've achieved sobriety through AA, meetings offer a space to share experiences, provide encouragement and work through the 12 steps.

The anonymity of AA members is highly respected and considered a fundamental principle of the organisation. This anonymity protects individuals' privacy and fosters an environment of trust and openness, allowing members to share their experiences and struggles without fear of judgement or repercussion.

One of the hallmark features of AA is the sponsorship system, where experienced members (sponsors) mentor newcomers through the 12-step process, offering guidance, support and accountability. This one-on-one relationship plays a crucial role in helping individuals navigate the challenges of early recovery and build a strong foundation for long-term sobriety.

In addition to regular meetings and sponsorship, AA literature, including the 'Big Book' (Alcoholics Anonymous) and the 'Twelve Steps and Twelve Traditions', serves as an essential resource for members to deepen their understanding of the programme and its principles.

Overall, AA provides a supportive community and a structured approach to recovery for individuals grappling with alcohol addiction. Its effectiveness and widespread acceptance have made it a cornerstone of addiction treatment worldwide, offering hope and assistance to millions of individuals seeking freedom from the grips of alcoholism.

Pros and Cons of Alcoholics Anonymous

AA has helped many people achieve sobriety. However, it also has features that may not work for everyone's needs, and it is reported to have only a 5–10% long term success rate (NPR Staff, 2014).

Pros

Below are some key advantages commonly associated with the program:

Peer Support

As an egalitarian ('belief in or advocacy for equality among all individuals') community of those facing alcohol dependence, AA provides judgement-free understanding and camaraderie. Members bond through shared hopes, struggles and victories along the recovery journey. This peer support system offers social motivation, a sense of belonging and inspiration to persevere. Just knowing others are walking parallel paths brings consolation.

Twelve-Step Programme

AA outlines a structured pathway to sobriety through its 12-step programme focused on self-reflection, surrender and restitution. By methodically working through each milestone with sponsor guidance tailored to their needs, members systematically confront addiction's complex personal roots before rebuilding independent sober lives.

Anonymity

Member anonymity promotes uninhibited sharing – crucial for healing deep emotional wounds that elicit shame if exposed. By guaranteeing confidentiality within groups, AA creates space for honest inventories of harmful behaviours and their motivations without fear of stigma. This vulnerability breeds accountability.

Sponsorship

AA's one-on-one sponsorship programme enables personal mentorship from experienced members. By supporting newcomers through turbulent periods, sponsors lead by example that the programme can work if applied consistently. Their empathy steadies resolve.

Spiritual Growth

In AA, people are encouraged to seek support from a 'higher power', without needing to follow any specific religion. This spiritual aspect helps individuals find meaning beyond alcohol. By letting go of their own desires and embracing humility, they can grow spiritually.

Regular Meetings

AA meetings offer regular community support to strengthen resolve and provide encouragement during difficult times. Sharing successes together fosters hope, with members serving as living examples of recovery. These meetings combat the sometimes isolating effects of addiction.

Personal Accountability

The programme fosters taking personal responsibility for errors and making living amends to those harmed. This brand of humility, restraint and penitence seeds positive growth.

Long-Term Sobriety Success Stories

The visible success of long-time AA members shows that AA works for keeping recovery strong. Their stories inspire new members to keep going through tough times, knowing that better days are ahead.

Inclusive Atmosphere

AA is a welcoming community that embraces diversity, bringing together people from all backgrounds who share a common struggle with alcoholism. In this supportive environment focused on healing, members freely contribute, bound together by compassion.

Accessibility

With so many meetings globally, AA offers consistent support for members relocating or travelling. Virtual meetings also increase accessibility – anyone can join anytime from anywhere.

Cons

Below are some key criticisms commonly associated with the program:

Spiritual Emphasis

AA's focus on a 'higher power' helps many but poses challenges for those with non-traditional beliefs. It conflicts with secular views and evidence-based approaches to recovery. For atheists or agnostics, this requirement may deter involvement, as the core of AA's practice revolves around submission to a higher authority. This could create a barrier for non-believers, limiting their access to needed support.

Focus on Powerlessness

The requirement that newcomers admit powerlessness conflicts with methodologies seeking to boost self-efficacy by exercising personal agency (an individual's ability to take action). As therapy often aims to foster an internal locus of control and self-actualisation, AA's emphasis on surrendering autonomy to an external higher authority contradicts this ethos for transformation. The deficit-focused framing needed in step one also risks embedding counterproductive thought patterns that reinforce notions of helplessness versus resilience. Those pursuing growth models seeking empowerment and positive psychology constructs emphasise assets not weaknesses – an incompatible perspective on change. By initially foregrounding surrender over action before building efficacy, buy-in becomes unlikely from this camp.

One-Size-Fits-All Approach

The structured 12-step programme lacks flexibility, so it is unable to tailor guidance to individual needs. This can be particularly challenging for those with additional diagnoses like depression or PTSD. Without the ability to adapt to individual complexities, AA may not offer comprehensive support. Additionally, the prescribed monolithic system may conflict with personal values of autonomy and self-actualisation. Few choices exist besides total acceptance of or departure from the doctrine.

Lack of Professional Therapy

AA, as a volunteer support group rather than a licensed clinical program, offers peer counselling rather than professional expertise. Individuals with complex needs requiring specialised therapies or psychiatric medications may find AA's non-professional environment insufficient. Co-occurring disorders and psychological traumas often accompany addiction, necessitating integrated professional treatment plans that include social support, which AA lacks. Therefore, individuals needing psychiatric medications or trauma-focused treatments like cognitive behavioural therapy (CBT) may struggle to complement AA with vital clinical care. This gap leaves vulnerable groups without adequate resources unless they seek separate fee-based help.

Anonymity Challenges

While anonymity is essential for open sharing in AA, breaches can occur in closely connected communities, particularly in remote rural areas or demographic networks where roles are intertwined. These breaches, along with lingering stigma around addiction, may discourage participation. Individuals hesitant to reveal their alcoholism to employers, family or friends may resist sharing even anonymously. Thus, the reliance on confidentiality within AA may falter without adequate protections, creating a catch-22 for certain individuals.

Reliance on Meetings

Regular attendance at in-person meetings is crucial for success in AA, but this can be difficult for individuals without reliable transportation or facing other barriers. While virtual meetings offer an alternative, they require technology skills and access to devices, excluding those without digital literacy or equipment. Moreover, meeting times may not accommodate individuals with unpredictable work schedules, hindering their ability to commit consistently. AA's emphasis on group sharing without flexible options may exclude those unable to attend regularly. While alternatives exist, many barriers to participation persist due to inflexibility.

No Formal Research Basis

AA's principles are based solely on the personal experiences of its founders rather than formal scientific research on addiction treatment effectiveness. This faith-based approach contrasts with evidence-based medicine advocates who view 12-step programmes overall as pseudoscientific, with no hard statistics validating success rates compared to control groups. No mechanisms currently exist demanding AA collect concrete data quantifying specific member outcomes. Without concrete data on its effectiveness compared to other methods, questions remain about AA's measurable impact.

Criticisms of Effectiveness

While AA provides irrefutable anecdotal stories of positive transformation, some longitudinal studies (observational research tracking subjects over time) suggest only 5–10% (NPR Staff, 2014) maintain total abstinence long-term – far below most evidence-backed interventions. This raises concerns about its overall effectiveness. Addiction is complex and requires customised solutions, so AA's uniform approach may not suit everyone. However, research shows that combining AA with professional therapy improves success rates, highlighting the value of integrated care (Moos & Moos, 2006). Quantitative critiques also overlook the qualitative community benefits of empowering human change through compassion and understanding. So, while AA may help some, relying solely on it may not address all aspects of addiction; personalised support combining clinical and peer resources may be more effective for some individuals.

Option 2: Cold Turkey

Going 'cold turkey' refers to the abrupt and complete cessation of alcohol consumption without any gradual reduction or tapering off. It involves stopping drinking suddenly and entirely. Quitting cold turkey is often a self-directed approach, where the person makes a conscious decision to stop drinking without professional intervention or a formal treatment programme.

Quitting alcohol abruptly through sheer determination can feel like the only option when desperation peaks. The concept often appeals to those craving immediate change from dependence. This section explores the realities people face when attempting to stop drinking on their own immediately.

Pros and Cons of the Quit Drinking Cold Turkey Approach

While the 'solo' and self-directed nature of this approach is attractive, anyone with a long-term habit of drinking alcohol, for whom a drink or several is more than a casual and occasional occurrence, will most likely struggle to go cold turkey without additional physical, mental, emotional and moral support from suitable sources. Professional medical care is absolutely essential for anyone with a high alcohol intake. In fact, be sure to check with your medical practitioner if you plan to attempt this.

Let's break it down.

Pros

Immediate Action and Increased Motivation

Taking immediate action, by making a decisive and instant commitment to an alcohol-free life, can be profoundly empowering, particularly for those ready for rapid change. The immediacy of this decision can be a significant motivator, strengthening a person's resolve and fostering determination to overcome the drinking habit. It's even possible to feel a somewhat euphoric sense of freedom and liberation from the dependence on the drinking habit.

Clear Break

Quitting abruptly provides a clear break from the habit of drinking, which some people find helps them mentally and emotionally move past their reliance on alcohol. It's a mark in the sand.

Rapid Detoxification

A clear break from daily drinking sessions allows for a quicker detoxification process compared to gradual tapering. The body starts eliminating alcohol and its by-products, so withdrawal symptoms and cravings may possibly subside sooner.

Potential for Quick Results

It's possible to experience relatively quick improvements in physical health, mental clarity and overall wellbeing once a change to an alcohol-free lifestyle has been made.

Self-Directed Independence

A person can feel empowered by making their own decision independently without necessarily relying on external sources. Since ultimately our choices for our health are our own responsibility, this is a beneficial attitude to have.

Cost-Effective

Compared to formal treatment programmes, this approach doesn't involve the expenses associated with professional interventions or rehabilitation centres.

Avoidance of Gradual Reduction Challenges

Some people find it challenging to adhere to gradual reduction plans. Going cold turkey eliminates the need for complex tapering schedules, making it a simpler approach.

Personal Transformation

A snap, final decision to quit drinking can be the start of a profound personal transformation. It can be a catalyst for a person to re-evaluate their lifestyle, make positive changes and develop new habits.

Cons

Potential for Intense Physical Withdrawal Symptoms and Serious Health Risks

Quitting abruptly can lead to intense withdrawal symptoms, including anxiety, insomnia, tremors, nausea and, in severe cases, seizures. The severity of symptoms can be overwhelming and may require medical attention. For people who are heavy drinkers or have been drinking for a long time, sudden withdrawal can lead to dangerous complications, including delirium tremens (DTs), which is a severe and potentially life-threatening condition. Always seek medical advice before quitting suddenly – this approach is not advisable for people with extreme reliance on alcohol (Schuckit et al., 2006).

Increased Risk of Relapse

The severity of withdrawal symptoms, persistent cravings and difficulty of habit change can increase the chance of returning to drinking. Research indicates that people who quit drinking cold turkey were more prone to relapse in the first few weeks. However, those who were able to stay abstinent for a month were more likely to remain abstinent for a year. This suggests that the initial period after quitting cold turkey is crucial, and people may need additional support during this time (Miller et al., 2001).

Managing Psychological Challenges and Mental Health Impact

Abruptly quitting alcohol can present psychological challenges such as mood swings, irritability and heightened stress, alongside impacting mental health with increased anxiety, depression and stress. Without proper support from experienced professionals that addresses both physical and psychological needs, navigating these difficulties can be particularly challenging and may increase the risk of returning to alcohol as a coping mechanism.

Lack of Professional Guidance

Going cold turkey as a self-directed approach lacks the structured guidance provided in professional treatment programmes. Without professional support, people may miss out on coping strategies and therapeutic assistance that can be greatly beneficial for maintaining abstinence.

Doesn't Consider the Whole Person

Alcohol intake, in any quantity, depletes the body of essential nutrition. In order to successfully transition to an alcohol-free life, the body needs to be restored to feel good. Simply cutting out alcohol without supporting the body's systems is likely to make the choice to remain alcohol-free unnecessarily difficult.

Research has found that people who quit drinking cold turkey experienced more severe withdrawal symptoms than those who gradually reduced their alcohol intake. However, they also found that these people were more likely to remain abstinent in the long term. This suggests that while quitting cold turkey can be challenging, it may also be more effective in the long run (Becker, 2012).

So, while some people may successfully quit drinking cold turkey, it's crucial to recognise the potential drawbacks and very real dangers. Seeking professional advice and care is recommended for those with a high regular alcohol intake and severe dependence.

Option 3: Willpower

Willpower, often referred to as self-control or self-discipline, is the ability to resist short-term temptations or impulses in order to achieve long-term goals or adhere to standards or values. In the context of giving up drinking alcohol, willpower refers to the mental strength and determination a person has to resist the urge to consume alcohol and to maintain an alcohol-free life. It means making a conscious and intentional decision to abstain from drinking, even when faced with triggers, cravings or social situations that may tempt the person to indulge.

Relying on willpower to give up drinking involves:

- exercising self-control over one's actions and choices

- making a firm decision to change a behaviour

- resisting triggers that may prompt the desire to drink, such as stress, social pressure or emotional challenges

- being goal-oriented – the goal serving as a constant motivator to stay focused on the positive outcomes of abstaining from alcohol

- possessing or building mental strength – the ability to navigate difficult situations without turning to alcohol

- mindfulness of one's thoughts, emotions and actions

As you will have surely thought by now, willpower and any other method for quitting alcohol are not 'mutually exclusive', and willpower does not actually stand alone. Willpower – to a greater or lesser extent – plays a part in any habit change and every quit drinking method. We've separated out willpower to address it individually, because understanding the pros and cons of relying on it is powerful knowledge.

Pros and Cons of Willpower

When trying to quit drinking, using personal willpower can seem like the way to go it alone. Just decide firmly to resist cravings and power through it solo. But while determination and willpower helps, it has real limitations too.

Pros

Independence and Flexibility

Relying on willpower means you manage the choice to stop drinking by yourself, not needing outside programmes or apps to help you stay alcohol-free. This gives you the flexibility to create a personal plan that fits your life and your goals for getting healthy on a timeline that works for you.

Intrinsic Motivation and Ownership

Using willpower taps into the inner motivations you already have inside you to make positive changes, instead of outside pressure. It puts you at the centre of the alcohol-free journey, making it feel like your choice instead of something you 'have to' do. This makes you more dedicated to stay stopped.

Self-Discipline and Responsibility

As we'll see in 'Cons' below, the strength of a person's willpower usually declines over the course of a day due to depletion. However, it can be restored or replenished through rest, relaxation and activities that replenish mental energy, such as mindfulness meditation or taking breaks. Additionally, some evidence suggests that willpower can be strengthened through practice and training, similar to how a muscle can be developed (Audiffren et al., 2022). So, building up willpower takes work — it means getting better at self-control and sticking to what you choose even when it's hard. But as your discipline grows, so does your belief you can meet goals like alcohol-free living. You feel more responsible for making choices that help future you.

Personal Development

Relying on willpower not only fosters personal growth by navigating the challenges of quitting drinking but also contributes to building mental resilience. This journey encourages self-reflection, the development of coping mechanisms and — ideally — exploration of healthier lifestyle choices. Simultaneously, the conscious decision to rely on willpower enhances decision-making skills, empowering individuals to navigate situations and stressors without resorting to alcohol. This holistic approach to personal development is a key benefit of using willpower to achieve and sustain an intentional alcohol-free lifestyle.

Long-Term Empowerment

Once you do something challenging like quitting drinking with willpower, your confidence and belief in yourself will continue beyond that first achievement. It lifts you up so you feel in charge of your life path as an ongoing personal value and habit.

Cons

Limited Resource

Willpower is a finite resource that can be depleted over time through use. This phenomenon is often referred to as 'ego depletion'. Just like a muscle becomes fatigued with use, the exertion of self-control can deplete one's reserves of willpower. Studies have shown that engaging in tasks that require self-control can lead to a decrease in performance on subsequent tasks that also require self-control. For example, resisting the temptation to eat unhealthy food may reduce one's ability to focus on a difficult task later in the day (Audiffren et al., 2022). Willpower appears to consume energy in the brain, specifically in areas associated with self-control and decision-making, and prolonged exertion can lead to mental fatigue. So, chances are, your willpower may leave you high and dry, just when you need it most.

Unlikely to Address the Root Cause

Aside from the physical or chemical dependence that occurs with regular alcohol intake, dependence on the habit to provide distraction or relief from underlying emotional or mental issues is often at play. If underlying issues are indeed the root causes of problem drinking, willpower won't resolve those issues.

Limited Coping Mechanisms and Mental Strain

Without a good understanding of how to manage tough times and a plan for navigating the inevitable challenges that accompany changing any deeply ingrained habit, relying solely on willpower may result in limited coping mechanisms for stress, triggers and emotional challenges. This places a heavy burden on a person's mental strength. Depending solely on willpower to overcome intensely strong subconscious programming can be mentally exhausting, increasing the risk of succumbing to cravings and potentially resulting in lapses in self-control over the long term.

Vulnerability to Triggers and Risk of Relapse During Stress

With underlying emotional and mental challenges left unaddressed, willpower alone may be insufficient to navigate complex triggers and situations that contribute to problem drinking. High-stress situations can test the limits of willpower, and without appropriate coping strategies and support, individuals may be more susceptible to relapse when faced with intense stressors.

Potential for Negative Self-Image

A strong reliance on willpower may lead individuals to blame themselves if they experience setbacks or relapses. This negative self-image can hinder progress and perpetuate the cycle of problem drinking, as evident in many discussions in online sober support community forums.

Overemphasis on Individual Effort

An exclusive focus on willpower omits the benefits of external support, which can be crucial in the process of habit change. Individuals relying solely on willpower may lack a built-in support system, including the peer support found in group therapy or support groups. Recognising the need for help, seeking guidance and fostering social connections can be crucial for long-term abstinence.

Understanding the limits and dynamics of willpower can help individuals manage their self-control more effectively, by prioritising important tasks earlier in the day when willpower reserves are typically higher and taking breaks or engaging in activities that replenish mental energy when feeling depleted. Not that this helps when 5 p.m. rolls around... So, while willpower is a valuable aspect of abstaining from drinking, the complexity of dependence on alcohol means a multifaceted approach that addresses the physical, mental and emotional systems will likely be far more successful. Willpower alone may not be sufficient for everyone, especially in cases of severe alcohol dependence where medical intervention and more comprehensive treatment programmes may be necessary.

Option 4: Vitamin Therapy

The book *The Vitamin Cure for Alcoholism* explores using nutritional supplements to address addiction. It was co-authored by psychiatrist Dr Abram Hoffer and nutritionist Andrew W. Saul.

The approach focuses on orthomolecular medicine – using optimal amounts of nutrients like vitamins and minerals to maintain health. The authors provide insights on how this nutritional therapy can support people struggling with alcohol dependence.

Interestingly, AA co-founder Bill W. found niacin (vitamin B3) therapy so helpful to his own recovery that he wrote pamphlets encouraging other AA members to try it. Hundreds ended up recovering with niacin's aid. However, this nutritional treatment did not stick as an integral part of AA over time or become mainstream in addiction medicine.

Research shows those with heavy alcohol intake often have significant vitamin deficiencies. Studies link chronic drinking to lowered levels of vitamins B1, B3, B6, B9, A and E as well as magnesium, zinc and selenium (Hoyumpa, 1986). This nutrient depletion causes brain function changes that can perpetuate addiction.

Replenishing vitamins through supplements coupled with quitting alcohol may alleviate these deficiencies. Restoring nutrition provides stability and sound judgement that supports resisting relapse. Research indicates this nutritional correction could counteract cravings and withdrawal side effects (Hoyumpa, 1986).

While more studies are needed, preliminary findings suggest nutritional therapy holds promise for boosting recovery odds by redressing the chemical imbalances created by alcohol. Integrative treatments personalise support.

Adopting vitamin therapy as part of a quitting alcohol journey is not going to be of interest to everyone. But for those who have an interest in nutrition and doing things naturally, we think it's essential to know this information is out there!

Pros and Cons of Vitamin Therapy

The use of orthomolecular treatment, or vitamin therapy, for alcoholism and quitting drinking is a topic that has been explored by proponents of alternative and complementary medicine. While the scientific community may not universally endorse these approaches, some potential advantages have been suggested by advocates. As always, it's noteworthy that individual responses can vary, and any treatment decisions should be made in consultation with a healthcare professional.

Now we'll look closely at how vitamin-based treatment could both assist and fall short when managing alcohol dependence.

Pros

Nutrient Support

The idea behind vitamin therapy is providing nourishing substances like vitamins and minerals at optimal levels to help restore wellbeing. Supplementing aims to correct potential deficiencies caused by heavy drinking that may leave bodies feeling depleted or unwell.

Brain Health

Some B vitamins support brain cell functioning – important when alcohol has disrupted key processes, cognition and mood regulation. As changes occur when coming off alcohol, replenishing nutrients aids mental clarity and stable thinking by assisting neurological recovery.

Reduced Cravings

Some have found vitamin B3, or niacin, useful in easing alcohol cravings specifically as the body adjusted during early abstinence. This therapy did not necessarily enter addiction treatment protocols, but it still offers an affordable supplement that potentially smooths out transition periods for some.

Cellular Repair

Antioxidants are nutrients that help repair cell damage from internal wear and tear. Alcohol toxins cause substantial oxidative stress, likely contributing to frequent drinkers feeling unwell over time even if physical liver issues don't arise. Correcting this environment at the subcellular level through nutritional support may alleviate residual discomfort or fatigue during recovery.

Withdrawal Symptom Relief

Transitioning from physically depending on alcohol to sobriety can be aided by a comprehensive approach to nutrition that stabilises mood, digestion, sleep and cognition in an integrated way. Individual supplements like B vitamins and magnesium may address select withdrawal symptoms like anxiety, muscle tension or restlessness as well. Nutritional balancing carefully guides the body's resilience.

Of course, vitamin therapy alone cannot resolve entrenched behavioural and psychological drivers of addiction. But consciously restoring health from various angles empowers and supports those undertaking the somewhat formidable journey of freeing themselves from alcohol's grasp.

Cons

Lack of Scientific Consensus

Unlike other addiction treatments, vitamin therapy lacks large-scale studies proving effectiveness, so is controversial in mainstream medicine. While some feel it helps them personally, the scientific community at large remains sceptical about consistent results.

Individual Variability

As with most areas of health, vitamin needs and responses vary widely person-to-person based on genetics, lifestyle and stage of recovery. Standard protocols get tricky when something that helps one individual may not benefit others equally. Personalisation often requires trial and error.

Potential Safety Issues

Megadosing particular vitamins potentially carries some risk if people self-prescribe incorrectly or don't consider interactions with medications or health conditions. Working closely with medical professionals is a wiser choice.

Delaying Comprehensive Care

Vitamin therapy alone cannot address psychological, behavioural and social drivers fuelling addiction. While nutritional optimisation aids overall wellness, solely relying on it risks postponing more holistic care like counselling, group support and lifestyle changes that sustain freedom from alcohol dependence long-term after the initial detox stages.

Financial Commitment

Out-of-pocket costs can limit accessibility to vitamin-based treatments since health insurance companies won't cover unproven approaches. Quality professional-grade supplements are expensive, so financial constraints exclude many without sufficient disposable income.

Risks of Self-Treatment

People understandably want affordable, accessible solutions, leading them to self-prescribe vitamin regimens after internet searches. But attempting this without seeking medical guidance could pose risks. Ideally, individuals would work closely with a trusted medical practitioner to ensure a safe and effective approach to vitamin therapy. However, with limited buy-in from the mainstream medical community, this support may not be forthcoming.

In summary, the lack of rigorous evidence on nutritional therapy protocols for addiction recovery poses uncertainties around consistency and safety when adopting this approach. Certainly, research it for yourself and consider the beneficial messages, but always consult with healthcare professionals before making decisions about self-administering medications – whether they be naturally occurring, or not.

Option 5: Medication-Assisted Treatment

Medication-assisted treatment (MAT) is an evidence-based approach to treating AUD that involves the use of approved medications, in combination with counselling and behavioural therapies, to provide a comprehensive treatment plan. The medications used in MAT for AUD include disulfiram, which creates an unpleasant reaction when alcohol is consumed; naltrexone, which reduces cravings and blocks the pleasurable effects of alcohol; and acamprosate, which helps restore balance to brain chemistry disrupted by chronic heavy drinking. Treatment plans are individualised based on a patient's specific needs and response to the medications, with healthcare providers assessing the severity of the addiction and any co-occurring disorders to tailor the optimal combination of medication, counselling and other supports.

Pros and Cons of Medication-Assisted Treatment

Pros

Research-Backed Effectiveness

Extensive studies have shown that MAT, when combined with counselling and behavioural therapies, can be highly effective in treating AUD, improving treatment outcomes and long-term recovery rates (Robertson et al., 2018).

Reduced Cravings and Withdrawal Symptoms

The medications used in MAT help reduce alcohol cravings, alleviate withdrawal symptoms and block the rewarding effects of alcohol, providing important physiological support during recovery.

Improved Treatment Adherence and Outcomes

MAT helps improve adherence to treatment, reduces the risk of relapse and can be used as part of a long-term maintenance strategy to sustain recovery over time.

Integrated Approach

By combining medication with counselling and therapy, MAT addresses both the physical and psychological components of addiction in a comprehensive manner.

Individualised Treatment

MAT allows treatment to be tailored to each individual's unique needs, goals and response to medications, optimising outcomes.

Improved Quality of Life

MAT has been shown to improve treatment engagement, reduce alcohol-related problems, increase quality of life and lower the risk of relapse and overdose compared to treatments without medication.

Cons

Potential Side Effects

The medications used in MAT can cause side effects in some people, ranging from mild (nausea, headache, dizziness) to more severe, depending on the specific medication.

Stigma and Hesitance

Some people may be hesitant to take medications for AUD treatment due to the stigma associated with using drugs to treat addiction or a preference for abstinence-only approaches.

Adherence Risk

There is a potential risk of non-adherence to the medication regimen, which would reduce its effectiveness.

Cost and Accessibility Limitations

MAT may involve limitations in terms of cost and accessibility, depending on an individual's insurance coverage and treatment setting.

Potential Drug Interactions

There is a potential for drug interactions with MAT medications, which must be carefully managed by healthcare providers.

Variable Effectiveness

While MAT can be highly effective, it may not work for everyone with AUD, as treatment outcomes can vary based on individual factors such as the severity of the addiction and co-occurring disorders.

Potential for Over-Reliance or Dependence on Medication

Depending on the individual and the treatment plan, there's a risk of relying too heavily on medication without addressing the underlying behavioural, psychological and psychosocial aspects of addiction and alcohol use through counselling and therapy. Some would say that complementary counselling and behavioural therapies are essential for a comprehensive approach.

Risk of Continued Drinking

While MAT can significantly reduce cravings and support abstinence, it does not guarantee that individuals won't drink. Some people may still consume alcohol.

MAT is an evidence-based, integrated treatment approach that has helped many people with AUD achieve and sustain recovery by addressing both the physiological and psychological aspects of addiction. While there are potential drawbacks to consider, such as side effects and cost limitations, MAT is a valid option that expands access to effective care for alcohol addiction when combined with behavioural treatments and tailored to individual needs. Open communication with qualified healthcare providers is essential for determining if MAT is an appropriate choice and optimising its effectiveness.

Option 6: Guidance Through Coaching, Counselling or Therapy

Embarking on the journey to quit drinking can be greatly supported by enlisting the assistance of a suitably qualified and experienced coach, counsellor or therapist. Such a person offers you invaluable insights, guidance, support and accountability tailored to address your specific needs and challenges.

Coaching is a collaborative and goal-oriented process and typically focuses on the present and future. A trained and certified coach serves as your ally in identifying and working towards personal aspirations, providing unwavering support, motivation and accountability to keep you on track. Many coaches have extensive self-development backgrounds and may even draw from direct experience of the very challenges you are confronting, bringing unique insights and empathy to their practice. After all, some of us find our calling in coaching as a means to help others navigate the battles we ourselves have conquered!

Therapists and counsellors are trained professionals who can provide strategies and techniques to deal with cravings, teach skills for managing stress without alcohol, help repair damaged relationships and address underlying mental health issues that may be contributing to alcohol use. In the USA, UK, Australia and many other countries around the world, there is a wide range of therapists and counsellors available who specialise in addiction recovery. These include psychologists, social workers, licensed professional counsellors (LPCs), marriage and family therapists (MFTs), addiction counsellors and psychiatrists, among others.

So, if you're struggling with problem drinking, you may like to consider seeking out a suitable coach, counsellor or therapist to work with – one whom you feel hears you, you can relate to and you know has a track record in helping people with similar challenges to those you are dealing with.

Pros and Cons of Coaching, Counselling or Therapy

As with embarking on any new endeavour, it's helpful to understand the benefits and potential pitfalls before you begin.

Pros

There are many possible advantages of seeking intelligent guidance, one on one, with an empathetic, experienced and attentive individual. Here's a few to contemplate:

Personalised Support

One-on-one guidance provides tailored assistance based on an individual's unique circumstances, needs and goals. This approach ensures that the support received is relevant and targeted to the specific challenges and aspirations of the person seeking help.

Moral Support

Working with a dedicated professional offers emotional encouragement and understanding, fostering a sense of not being alone in the journey. This moral support can be invaluable in navigating the challenges and setbacks that may arise during the process of quitting drinking.

Accountability

Regular check-ins and goal-setting with a professional can help ensure commitment and progress. Having someone to report to and share successes and struggles with can provide a strong sense of accountability, motivating individuals to stay on track.

Insights Into Emotional Wellbeing

One-on-one sessions offer a safe space with opportunities for self-reflection and gaining insights into behaviours, triggers, patterns and deeper emotional wounds that may be contributing to drinking as a form of self-medication. Exploring and addressing these underlying emotional issues can be crucial for long-term recovery and emotional healing.

Coping Strategies and Guidance for Calmness

Experienced professionals can provide techniques, strategies and effective coping mechanisms for people to manage stress, anxiety and triggers without resorting to alcohol. Learning and practising these skills under guidance can help individuals develop an essential toolkit for maintaining calmness and resilience in the face of challenges.

Neuroplasticity and Brain Rewiring

Therapeutic techniques utilised in one-on-one sessions can facilitate the rewiring of neural pathways, promoting healthier habits and thought patterns. This process of neuroplasticity can support long-term changes in behaviour and emotional regulation.

Goal Achievement

Working with a professional allows for setting and working towards specific, achievable goals related to the choice to be alcohol-free. Having clear objectives and a plan of action can provide direction and motivation throughout the journey.

Holistic Approach

One-on-one guidance often takes a holistic approach, addressing physical, emotional and psychological aspects for a comprehensive approach to recovery. This multi-faceted perspective acknowledges the interconnectedness of various factors in the journey towards an alcohol-free life.

Confidentiality

One-on-one sessions provide a private and confidential space to discuss concerns and challenges openly. Knowing that any personal information shared will be kept confidential can create a sense of safety and trust, allowing for more honest and vulnerable conversations.

Professional Expertise

One-on-one guidance draws on the expertise of trained professionals – such as coaches, counsellors or therapists – who have experience in areas such as habits, thoughts, emotions, addiction and recovery. Access to this specialised knowledge and experience can be invaluable in navigating the complexities of quitting drinking.

Long-Term Success

One-on-one guidance aims to build a foundation for sustained abstinence from alcohol and overall wellbeing. By addressing underlying issues, developing coping strategies and fostering personal growth, this approach can support individuals in achieving long-term success in their alcohol-free journey.

Cons

There are potential disadvantages of seeking a one-on-one service to get help with quitting drinking. Here are some to consider:

Medical Record Implications

Engaging in one-on-one guidance, especially with licensed professionals, may result in a documented history of mental health or addiction issues in medical records. This can raise concerns about potential implications for future employment or insurance opportunities.

High Expenses

Sessions with professionals can be costly, especially if not covered by insurance. Financial constraints may limit access to this type of support or create additional stress for individuals seeking help.

Variation in Approach

Different professionals may have varying approaches and levels of effectiveness, leading to uncertainty in the outcome. It can be challenging to determine the best fit without trying multiple options, which can be time-consuming and expensive.

Limited Personal Understanding

While professional therapists and counsellors have academic knowledge, they may lack personal experience or a deep understanding of the emotional struggles associated with addiction. This can create a gap in empathy and relatability, potentially impacting the outcomes.

Admitting to a Stranger

Opening up about personal issues to someone unfamiliar, even if a trained professional, can evoke feelings of humiliation or shame. This emotional barrier may hinder the level of openness necessary for effective progress.

Communication Barriers

Individuals who are not naturally inclined to verbal communication may find it challenging to express their thoughts and feelings in a one-on-one setting. This can hinder the effectiveness of sessions.

Limited Availability

One-on-one sessions may have scheduling constraints and limited availability due to cost or availability factors. This can delay getting the help needed.

Compatibility in Therapeutic Relationships

The effectiveness of one-on-one guidance hinges greatly on the compatibility between the individual seeking help and the specific professional providing it. A good match fosters a strong alliance, enhancing the effectiveness of the coaching or therapy. However, if there are differences in cultural background or personal values, this can lead to a mismatch that affects levels of understanding, trust and comfort within the therapeutic relationship.

Lack of Peer Support

One-on-one approaches may not provide the same level of peer support and communal understanding found in group settings. The absence of shared experiences and encouragement from others in similar situations can be a drawback for some individuals.

Limited Perspective

Relying solely on one professional's perspective may limit exposure to a broader range of therapeutic techniques and ideas. This narrow focus can potentially overlook alternative approaches that may be beneficial for an individual's unique needs.

While one-on-one guidance offers numerous advantages, it's essential to consider these potential disadvantages when deciding on the best approach for seeking help in quitting drinking.

Option 7: Self-Help Books and Resources

Today, on the journey to an alcohol-free lifestyle, there is a broad spectrum of available resources beyond professional help. While 10 years ago I struggled to find so much as a single book to read to help me get to the bottom of what I was going through in trying to control my intake of alcohol, now options abound – we can explore the realm of 'quit lit', online courses and community support groups. There is a plethora of self-help books, educational platforms and virtual communities ready to provide insights, advice and ever-present moral support on the path to remaining alcohol-free.

Pros and Cons of Self-Help Books and Resources

Although a wealth of resources exists at our fingertips to aid in our alcohol-free future, amid this abundance there are opportunists and potential traps. It's crucial to approach with caution and discernment. Let's delve into the nuances.

Pros

Abundance of Published Books

There is a substantial number of self-help books addressing alcoholism and sobriety. According to estimates, there are thousands of books available, offering diverse perspectives, strategies and personal narratives. Options include physical books, ebooks and audiobooks, which are highly affordable and accessible for all. Look for those with a high number of good reviews; however, it's important to be discerning. Some books may have a high rating due to aggressive marketing tactics or because they push follow-up or 'back-end' products, which could compromise the integrity of the content. Additionally, certain books may contain outdated information or lack a broader perspective on the complexities of alcohol dependence. It's essential to critically evaluate the credibility and relevance of the information presented before choosing to follow any particular doctrine.

Diversity in Approaches and Accessibility of Resources

Available self-help methods provide a broad spectrum of approaches, ranging from books, blogs, online courses and mobile apps to telephone hotlines, in-person courses and community support groups. This diversity enables people to select resources that suit their preferences and needs, ensuring accessibility to a wide audience, whether they prefer digital or traditional methods.

Global Reach and Community Engagement in Online Sobriety Communities

The emergence of online sobriety communities, particularly on platforms like Facebook, has transcended physical boundaries. These virtual communities, estimated to number in the thousands, connect individuals worldwide and cater to diverse preferences. They offer gender-specific, age-specific and method-specific groups, fostering a sense of global support and understanding. This significant growth in online sobriety communities reflects a rich tapestry of shared experiences and varied paths to living without alcohol, contributing to a vibrant sense of community engagement among like-minded people.

Broadening Visibility, Embracing 'Sober Curious'

In recent years, the visibility of sobriety, alcoholism recovery and the alcohol-free lifestyle has expanded, fostering a more open and understanding societal conversation. This inclusivity extends to the 'sober curious' movement, reflecting a growing curiosity and acceptance of alternative paths to sobriety that is further enriching the discourse on recovery.

Global Participation in Alcohol-Free Challenges

Beyond individual efforts, international events like 'Dry July', 'Sober October' and 'Hello Sunday Morning' encourage a collective break from alcohol. These initiatives foster a sense of global camaraderie, providing individuals with structured challenges and shared goals for alcohol-free periods. Other notable events, such as 'Dry January' and 'Sober Spring', further contribute to the worldwide movement towards mindful and temporary abstinence from alcohol.

The Rise of On-Trend Alcohol-Free Drinks

The rise of craft breweries and distilleries focusing on alcohol-free drink options is not just a passing trend but a growing market segment with considerable potential – which also speaks volumes about consumer demand. People are becoming more health-conscious and seeking choices that allow them to enjoy socialising without the negative effects of alcohol. So, if you were to seek out some of these on-trend drink options, you would have the opportunity to actually be an alcohol-free trail blazer.

Cons

Of course, it's not all beer and skittles (oh look – a drinking reference in a common idiom!) and there are some shortcomings of the self-help approach to quitting drinking:

Varied Quality and Intent of Resources

The abundance of self-help resources brings the challenge of varying quality and potential biases, requiring people to discern and choose carefully among the available options. Well-reviewed books and courses are often good quality, but do keep an eye out for a possible agenda on the part of the publisher or author who is offering their own services to readers.

Potential Lack of Professional Guidance

Self-help methods will naturally lack the direct oversight and personalised guidance provided by professionals (coaches, counsellors, therapists), potentially leading to gaps in addressing complex individual needs.

Isolation and Limited Peer Support

Engaging primarily in self-help methods may result in a lack of the peer support and shared experiences found in group settings, potentially leading to feelings of isolation during the journey to becoming alcohol-free and beyond.

Risk for Individuals With High Dependency

For those with a high level of alcohol dependency, relying solely on self-help methods without close supervision by a medical professional poses significant risks. The absence of direct medical oversight could be dangerous, especially when dealing with severe withdrawal symptoms or complex medical conditions associated with prolonged alcohol use.

Option 8: A Holistic Approach to Lifestyle Transformation

We know from numerous scientific studies that alcohol dependence likely involves a complex interplay of genetic, neurobiological, emotional coping, habits and environmental factors. You might like to refer back to Chapter 2 where we looked at these factors in detail.

It makes sense, then, that to come up with the most successful approach to achieve an alcohol-free lifestyle, each of these factors needs to be adequately addressed.

So, that's what we will look at here – a holistic approach to the alcohol issue, taking into account all factors potentially at play for a person finding that being the one in charge in their relationship with alcohol is a challenge.

This is where the power is. When AA says 'we're powerless over alcohol', they're partially right. Acknowledging that we have multiple of these factors stacked up against us may make the task seem insurmountable. However, with knowledge, understanding and a determination to get more out of life, we can divide and conquer. We can look at each factor individually and work on ways to address them – in our favour.

Addressing Each Factor for Success

Addressing the Genetic Factor

I'm reminded of a saying by Steve Maraboli, 'Incredible change happens in your life when you decide to take control of what you do have power over instead of craving control over what you don't' (Maraboli, 2022).

If the genetic factor is at play, we can't do anything about it. We can't change our genes. If we do know of a genetic link, that provides a piece of information we can understand and use to make our decision about whether alcohol has a place in our life – or not.

Addressing the Neurobiological Factor

Removing alcohol allows the brain and body to heal and reduces dependence and cravings. (This may require medical supervision for long-term or heavy drinkers.) Cravings will reduce over time but for some may still be not too far from the surface, and for some they can return unexpectedly even after many months. So, tactics need to be employed to anticipate and manage them. Here are some quick tips for managing alcohol cravings:

- **Identify triggers:** Know what prompts your cravings, like stress or certain environments.

- **Develop coping strategies:** Find activities or techniques to deal with cravings, like exercise, helpful thought processes or relaxation methods.

- **Seek support:** Surround yourself with supportive people who understand your journey.

- **Stay distracted:** Engage in fulfilling activities that take your mind off cravings, like hobbies or spending quality time with friends or family.

- **Consider therapy or coaching:** Explore therapies like CBT to address underlying issues. Interview potential coaches who have walked a mile in your shoes.

- **Take care of yourself:** Prioritise sleep, nutrition and exercise for overall well-being.

- **Stay active:** Engage in meaningful activities that bring joy and fulfilment.

- **Stay vigilant:** Understand that cravings may return, so be prepared and proactive in managing them.

By having these strategies as part of your life, you can learn to effectively manage cravings and maintain an alcohol-free lifestyle.

Addressing the Environmental Factor

Navigating the environmental influences of family, friends, society, culture and advertising is crucial for success. Recognising these pressures is the first step. Remembering your *'why'* for quitting is paramount – because true success hinges on prioritising personal wellbeing over societal norms and marketing tactics. To resist the allure of alcohol, focus on the positive aspects of an alcohol-free lifestyle, stay committed to your reasons for quitting and embrace the benefits and freedom that comes with this decision.

Addressing the Emotional Coping Factor

Many turn to alcohol to cope with emotional distress such as stress, anxiety or trauma. While it may provide temporary relief, alcohol ultimately compounds rather than resolves these issues. Overindulgence in alcohol, along with other behaviours (over-eating, gambling, gaming, shopping and the like), serves as a distraction or coping mechanism for underlying emotional discomfort. Recognising these patterns is crucial in breaking free from harmful coping mechanisms and beginning to address emotional struggles effectively with a coach, therapist or counsellor.

Addressing the Habitual Factors

We prepare dinner, we have a drink. It's 5 p.m., we have a drink. We have a glass of wine and some crackers and cheese. We're used to picking up a glass and drinking for various effects and also as a physical thing to do with our hands and our body. The ceremonial opening of the bottle and filling of the glass and drinking (perhaps with a significant other – Tony and I would do a 'cheers and a kiss', which became as ritualistic as the tea ceremony in Japan!) is a habit. What happens if we suddenly stop an ingrained habit? It's uncomfortable. Mighty uncomfortable. So, addressing this factor adds to the steep gradient of the mountain we're going to climb to stop drinking. We need to be alert to this and be ready to create new habits.

Here's how to address all these factors.

A Better Body Blueprint: Transformative Life Enriching Choices

What We Consume

We cannot expect to feel good if our body doesn't have the right type of fuel in it to perform well. Don't put lawnmower fuel in a racing car!

Hydration: Even mild dehydration can negatively impact mood, attention and brain function. Maintain water intake.

Nutrition: A well-nourished body is less likely to crave unhealthy substances. The gut microbiome, considered our 'second brain', significantly influences how we feel. Minimise (ideally eliminate) processed foods and eat whole foods.

Physical Activity

Keep moving: Being sedentary can contribute to feelings of depression and sluggishness. However, regular physical activity, including even a brief session of exercise, has been consistently linked to improved mood and reduced symptoms of depression and anxiety. Exercise releases feel-good chemicals in the brain, improves sleep quality, boosts confidence and acts as a potent stress reliever. Overall, staying active not only enhances physical health but also significantly contributes to mental wellbeing, providing a natural and effective way to lift our spirits and maintain a positive outlook on life.

Sleep

Sleep is as important as diet and exercise for everyday functioning — including mental health — as well as long-term health. Become an expert in the latest on sleep research by exploring the book *Why We Sleep* by Matthew Walker (2017).

Breathing

Breathing influences our mental wellbeing profoundly. By practising proper breathing techniques, such as nose breathing and deep diaphragmatic breathing, we can activate the parasympathetic nervous system, calm our minds and enhance mental focus. Additionally, correcting poor breathing habits supports various aspects of physical health, from improving lung function and digestion to reducing dependence on medications for conditions like asthma or anxiety. Become an expert in this topic by delving into the book *Breath* by James Nestor (2020).

Emotional Wellbeing

Mindfulness and meditation: Embracing these ago-old practices helps with mental wellbeing and resilience by reducing stress, improving emotions management and supporting a more positive outlook on life. Studies show that certain mindfulness practices lead to significant improvements in physical and psychological symptoms, while regular meditation increases resilience, helping people bounce back from adversity more quickly (Oh et al., 2022). Additionally, mindfulness boosts the body's immune function, improves relationships and can even change the brain's structure (in a good way!). Let go of the notion that this is for hippies – current science is highlighting the incredibly powerful impact of mindfulness and meditation on overall health and resilience.

Emotional freedom technique (EFT): Studies show that EFT (also known as 'tapping') reduces anxiety and improves physiological measures of health, providing a non-pharmaceutical option for managing anxiety and enhancing emotional and physical wellbeing. Additionally, EFT has been found to effectively reduce cravings for alcohol, suggesting its potential as a tool in alcohol addiction treatment. This technique, often called 'psychological acupressure', combines cognitive therapy and acupressure, offering a flexible approach that can be self-administered or guided by a professional to address various mental health issues, phobias and even physical pain (Church et al.,

2018). EFT's efficacy is gaining recognition in the scientific community, with the American Psychological Association recognising it as an evidence-based practice for specific phobias (Greenberg, 2017). Developed in the 1990s, EFT is growing in popularity as a holistic approach to emotional wellbeing, despite earlier views of it being 'alternative' or pseudoscience.

Cognitive behavioural therapy (CBT): CBT is a widely used form of psychotherapy with extensive research support, and is effective for treating various mental health conditions like depression, anxiety and substance use disorders. It can be effective in significantly reducing the frequency of heavy drinking in people with AUD. CBT works by helping a person recognise and change unhelpful thought patterns and behaviours. It's like reprogramming the brain to respond differently to the triggers that lead to excessive drinking.

Something to Do With Your Hands and Capture Your Interest

Engaging hobbies: Having absorbing, meaningful hobbies can provide a healthy distraction and alternative to drinking. Studies suggest that engaging hobbies can reduce the likelihood of alcoholism, improve mental health, provide social connections, boost happiness and productivity, enhance creativity and even increase longevity (Zhang et al., 2021).

An interesting anecdote: I recently came across a post in a backyard chicken keepers Facebook Group where a member shared that caring for her chickens motivated her to maintain an alcohol-free lifestyle. She wanted to be the best chicken mama possible!

Tracking and Accountability

Journalling: Keeping a journal or tracking progress can increase self-awareness, accountability and commitment to change. Research suggests that expressive writing and self-monitoring can be effective tools in reducing alcohol consumption and supporting recovery from alcohol dependence (Zhang et al., 2021).

Coaching or therapy: Working with a personal coach, success coach or therapist who understands your journey can provide invaluable support. Recovery coaches and personal coaching can significantly improve quitting drinking success rates, help develop coping strategies, enhance motivation and provide ongoing support.

Pros and Cons of Lifestyle Changes With Holistic Approaches

Here's what to consider when adopting lifestyle changes to support your alcohol-free future.

Pros

We can't overemphasise the benefits of making optimal lifestyle choices with an approach that looks after all of you as a human being! Here are the many benefits of this approach:

Addresses Root Causes

This approach tackles the underlying genetic, neurobiological, emotional and habitual factors that contribute to alcohol dependence. By addressing these root causes, rather than just the symptoms, this approach offers a more comprehensive and sustainable solution.

Empowers the Individual

By adopting strategies to nourish the body, manage emotions and develop new habits, people become empowered to take control of their own journey to an alcohol-free lifestyle. This approach equips people with the tools they need to abstain long term, rather than relying solely on external interventions.

Enhances Overall Health and Wellbeing

This approach focuses on optimising physical health through proper nutrition, hydration, exercise and sleep. These lifestyle changes not only support an alcohol-free lifestyle but also promote overall health and wellbeing, leading to improved quality of life.

Develops Emotional Resilience

Incorporating practices like mindfulness, meditation, EFT and CBT helps people develop emotional resilience. By learning to manage stress, anxiety and negative emotions in healthy ways, people are less likely to turn to alcohol as a coping mechanism.

Fosters Personal Growth

The process of overcoming alcohol dependence through lifestyle changes can be a profound journey of personal growth and self-discovery. As people develop new coping skills, build healthier habits and gain self-awareness, they often experience improvements in self-esteem, relationships and overall life satisfaction.

Flexible and Customisable

This approach can be tailored to each person's unique needs, preferences and circumstances.

Provides Long-Term Benefits

Unlike short-term interventions or quick fixes, a holistic lifestyle approach offers long-term benefits. By addressing the underlying issues and developing healthy coping mechanisms, people are better equipped to maintain their new lifestyle in the long run.

Encourages Self-Reflection and Mindfulness

Practices like journalling, tracking and mindfulness encourage self-reflection and increased self-awareness. This heightened understanding of one's thoughts, emotions and triggers can be invaluable in maintaining good mental health and managing emotions.

A Proactive Approach

Rather than simply reacting to life and succumbing to the consequences of alcohol dependence, a holistic lifestyle approach is proactive. By focusing on prevention and wellness, this approach empowers individuals to take charge of their health and wellbeing before problems escalate.

Cons

Realistically, these aren't downsides, as a lifestyle change that supports the whole person to be healthier is really the only way forward! Rather, think of this following list as potential areas that might trip you up or challenge you – and be ready for them before they do!

Requires Commitment and Effort

Adopting a holistic lifestyle approach requires significant commitment and effort. Changing deeply ingrained habits, developing new coping strategies and maintaining motivation can be challenging, especially in the face of triggers and setbacks.

May Be Time-Consuming

Implementing lifestyle changes, participating in support sessions and engaging in new activities can be time-consuming. Finding the time and energy to prioritise self-care and recovery amid other life responsibilities can be a challenge.

Can Be Emotionally Challenging

Confronting underlying emotional issues and learning new coping strategies can be emotionally taxing. The process of self-discovery and change can sometimes feel overwhelming or uncomfortable.

Requires Patience and Persistence

Lifestyle changes rarely produce overnight results. It can take time to experience the full benefits of a holistic approach and progress may be gradual.

May Require Professional Support

Depending on the severity of alcohol dependence and any co-occurring mental health issues, additional professional support may be necessary, bringing with it potential financial, geographical and time constraints.

Risk of Relapse

This approach aims to reduce the risk of relapse by addressing underlying issues, but the risk can never be eliminated entirely. Stressful life events, triggers or unexpected challenges happen, so ongoing vigilance and support are necessary.

Potential for Overwhelming Lifestyle Changes

The prospect of overhauling one's lifestyle, from diet and exercise to stress management and emotional coping, can feel overwhelming. The sheer scope of changes suggested may be daunting for some, leading to resistance or ambivalence.

Requires Self-Motivation

Personal accountability is paramount. While external support is important, ultimately the individual must take responsibility for their own recovery journey. This can be challenging for those who struggle with self-discipline or who are used to relying on external forces for motivation.

May Not Be Sufficient for Severe Cases

In cases of severe alcohol dependence or co-occurring mental health disorders, a holistic lifestyle approach alone may not be sufficient. Medical intervention, intensive treatment programmes or specialised care may be necessary in addition to lifestyle changes.

What to Do With This Information

In this chapter we have explored the various approaches and elements involved in quitting drinking, spelling out that there is no one-size-fits-all solution. Each method has its own unique benefits and drawbacks – or gaps – and the effectiveness of any given approach depends largely on an individual's specific needs, circumstances and personal preferences.

Reflect on this information thoughtfully, choosing elements that resonate with you and align with your goals. While considering the potential drawbacks we've discussed, arm yourself with awareness. Draw wisdom from the experiences of others and courageously forge ahead on your journey!

Author's note: You will no doubt have noticed that our list of strategies for quitting drinking does not include options like inpatient and outpatient treatment programmes and other not-for-profit and community-based programmes. There are two reasons for this. One reason is that we do not have first-hand experience of attending these types of programmes as they either were not available or we did not know of them. I did know about AA and went so far as looking them up in my area, but was never going to attend, for fear of someone knowing me if I did so! The second reason is that it's not realistically possible to cover all options available. The strategies we've covered here serve to highlight the critical elements to seek out to be sure you cover all the needs you will have on your journey. It's a place to start!

Feedback

Do you have particular insights into or experiences with these strategies that provide a more up-to-date light on the information we have provided here? What would you add? What would you disagree with? We invite you to share your views with us at feedback@organisedcoaching.com

Chapter 5:

When You Know You Need to Stop Drinking

Step 1: Realisation That There Is a Problem

If there was no problem, you wouldn't be here. My story is that I had tried to moderate my drinking for many years – probably over a decade – but never could for any significant length of time, except each time I was pregnant. Seemingly, I could make the decision to look after another person, but not to look after myself, despite knowing the amount I was drinking at times probably wasn't good for me!

The crazy thing is, I had *no concept* that *not* drinking was even an *option* for me! Such was the strength of the cultural and societal conditioning, I was always aiming to be a person who drank alcohol, just not too much. A person in control, who could moderate their intake. It simply never occurred to me that being a non-drinker was a valid choice. Looking back, I attribute that to the pervasive environmental influences around drinking.

The turning point for me was when the pain of not drinking (the 'fear of missing out') became less than the pain of the daily struggle to control the desire to drink. It suddenly became easy to give up. In fact, on the day I quit, I declared to myself: 'Just for *one* year. I'm not going to drink for *one* year.' The relief was enormous. And from three weeks in, feeling so much better and freed from that constant battle, I never looked back. The realisation that drinking was causing me more pain than pleasure was a crucial moment. It was the catalyst that allowed me to make a firm decision and stick to it.

So, what will it be for you? How will you decide your path forward from here?

Pertinent Questions to Contemplate

1. How often do you find yourself exceeding your intended limit when drinking? Consider this carefully. Do you set out to have just one glass but consistently end up having more? Be honest with yourself about your patterns.

2. Have you faced negative personal or professional consequences because of your drinking? Think about your day-to-day life. Have you called in sick to work because you were hungover? Have you missed important conference sessions after overindulging the night before? Have you felt unwell getting the kids to school after drinking too much? These are all red flags.

3. When trying to cut back, do you struggle to consistently stick to your limits? Government health departments recommend having a few alcohol-free days per week. Can you manage this, or do you find yourself drinking daily because abstaining is too hard? This is a sign that your drinking is becoming a dependency.

4. How does alcohol impact your physical and mental wellbeing? Do you often feel sick, unwell or hungover after drinking? Do you worry about your alcohol intake? Do you notice that emotional issues seem to worsen over time when you're drinking regularly?

5. Have loved ones expressed concern about your drinking habits? Sometimes those closest to us notice things before we're ready to admit them to ourselves. Have you noticed your partner, family or friends glancing at your glass as you pour

another drink, even if they don't say anything? They may be worried about you.

6. Have you noticed increased tolerance – needing more alcohol for the same effects? Tolerance is a clear sign that your body is adapting to alcohol. Think about times when you've had a period of abstinence. Do you initially feel satisfied with less alcohol, but within a month or two find yourself wanting to drink more to get the same 'buzz'?

7. How does alcohol use align with your personal values and long-term goals? Think carefully on this – and about the facts we've covered so far. Chapter 1 detailed alcohol's capabilities; Chapter 2 explained why people develop drinking problems; Chapter 3 looked at reasons for considering quitting. Now, consider your own drinking habits. Does your current alcohol use truly align with your values and goals? Or are you experiencing cognitive dissonance – the mental discomfort that arises when your beliefs and behaviours are in conflict?

8. Have you tried moderating your drinking before, and if so, what were the results? Many people try to cut back on their drinking before they consider quitting entirely. If you've tried this, how did it go? Were you able to easily take drink-free days each week? Could you take or leave alcohol without worry? Or did you feel agitated and go to great lengths to get the alcohol you wanted? Be honest about your past attempts.

9. How do you feel about the idea of abstaining from alcohol for a set period, like one month? Challenges like 'Dry January' or 'Sober October' have become popular in recent years. Have you ever attempted one of these? How does the thought of taking on such a challenge make you feel? Excited and motivated? Or filled with apprehension and dread? Your reaction can tell you a lot.

10. Can you envisage a positive, fulfilling life without relying on alcohol? I'll share something personal. I once held the belief that non-drinkers were unsophisticated. Having been raised in a family that appreciated 'fine' wines, I genuinely believed that

those who didn't drink were uneducated and less worldly than I was. I truly thought they were missing out on one of life's great pleasures. Looking back, I see how outrageous and misguided that belief was! It was a product of my conditioning and the alcohol-centric culture I was immersed in.

After contemplating these questions and honestly examining your responses, what are your thoughts? Perhaps alcohol is no big deal for you. You can take it or leave it and it doesn't occupy much space in your mind. Or perhaps your next drink is constantly on your mind and the idea of not indulging fills you with a sense of anxiety, or even panic.

If you find yourself relating more to the latter, it's likely that alcohol has become more of a problem than you'd like to admit.

Working through these questions and carefully considering your answers will provide valuable insight into where you stand on the 'should I drink or shouldn't I drink?' question. If many of your responses align with the problematic patterns and consequences associated with excessive drinking, it's a strong indication that quitting alcohol may be the healthiest choice for you.

But don't worry – recognising this is the first and most important step.

Remember, you're the only one who can make this decision and ensure its success. No one likes being told what to do, and lasting change comes from within. By honestly assessing your relationship with alcohol and its impact on your life, you're taking a brave and powerful step towards a healthier future.

In the next section, we'll explore the different options available to you and help you devise a personalised plan for moving forward on your unique journey with alcohol.

Step 2: Information Gathering, Decision Time and Action Time

By now, you've thoroughly contemplated the questions from Step 1 above and coupled that with the wealth of information provided in Chapters 1 to 4 of this book. At this point, you really have all the knowledge at your fingertips you are likely to need to make an informed decision about the role alcohol will play in your life moving forward.

Up until now, we have explored the pros and cons of drinking, giving you a balanced perspective on the potential benefits and drawbacks. Chapter 2 delved into the science of addiction, helping you understand the factors that can contribute to problematic drinking patterns. Chapter 3 encouraged you to consider your 'why' – your personal reasons for wanting to change your relationship with alcohol and the vision you have for your future. And Chapter 4 provided an overview of the various approaches to quitting drinking, highlighting how much the landscape has changed in just the past 5–10 years.

As you reflect on all this information, consider which points resonate most strongly with you. Do you recognise any of the risk factors for addiction in your own life? Do the cons of drinking outweigh the pros when you think about your long-term goals and values? Keep these insights in mind as you move into the decision-making phase.

Decision Time

Now it's time to get logical and strategic about your next steps. Based on everything you've learned and the self-reflection you've done, here are the three main options to consider:

Choice 1: Choose to Cut Back

If you believe that moderating your alcohol intake is a realistic and sustainable goal for you, then cutting back may be the right choice. However, it's important to be honest with yourself about your track record. Have you successfully cut back in the past? How long have you been trying to curb your drinking? If, like I had, you've been attempting moderation for years or even decades with little success, that's a strong indication that a more significant change may be necessary.

Choice 2: Choose to Abstain for Good

For those of us who find that even one drink can lead us back down the slippery slope to overindulgence, complete abstinence may be the wisest choice. If you've tried to moderate your drinking time and time again only to find yourself slipping back into old patterns, it might be time to consider giving up alcohol entirely. This can be a daunting prospect, but remember – countless people have successfully embraced an alcohol-free lifestyle and discovered a newfound sense of freedom and wellbeing.

You may be wondering how you'll cope without alcohol – don't worry, we'll address that in Step 3 below. For now, let's focus on synthesising the information you've gathered and using it to guide your decision-making process.

Choice 3: Choose to Abstain for a Set Period of Time

If the idea of never drinking again feels too overwhelming, consider committing to a set period of abstinence instead. This can be a great way to dip your toes into the alcohol-free waters and experience the benefits first-hand. Many people find that taking a break from drinking for a month or even a year provides valuable insights and helps them re-evaluate their relationship with alcohol. You might choose to abstain for 12 months and then reassess your decision at the end of that period. This is sometimes referred to as being 'sober curious' – a term that's gained popularity in recent years as more people experiment with temporary sobriety.

Action Time

Once you've made your decision, it's time to put it into action. In Chapter 6, we'll start working through the practical steps of implementing your choice, starting with grabbing a notebook or journal and writing down your 'why'. Having a clear and compelling reason for making this change will be invaluable in keeping you motivated and on track.

In addition, you'll start thinking about your support system. Who will be there to encourage and guide you along the way? Will you consider enlisting the help of a coach, therapist, counsellor or trusted friend who can provide accountability, support or advice when you need it most?

So, get ready to make a concrete plan.

But for now, in Step 3 below, we'll dive into the nitty-gritty of some of those nagging questions you'll have about navigating life without alcohol, from handling cravings to socialising sober. We'll get those answered before moving onto the plan.

Before we start, take a moment to celebrate the fact that you've made a decision and are taking action to create positive change in your life. You've got this!

Step 3: Managing the Decision Long-Term

Congratulations on making the life-affirming decision to rid your body of the alcohol toxin and reclaim your health, vitality and longevity! With a clearer head, more hours in the day and greater energy, your personal, business, entrepreneurial and experiential goals are more within reach than ever.

But now, a haze of questions will likely arise: What do I drink instead? What do I say when people ask why I'm not drinking? Does this mean I'll never have a drink again? How do I calm my nerves and cope with stress without alcohol?

Don't worry – we've got you covered. Here's our FAQ guide on how to manage your decision for the long haul.

What do I drink instead?

There's never been a better time to give up drinking! Mindfulness about alcohol consumption is on the rise, and more and more people are choosing to abstain. Plus, there are tons of delicious non-alcoholic alternatives available now.

Personally, I prefer to keep it simple with mineral water or soda water with a squeeze of lemon or lime. If I'm feeling fancy, I might opt for an 'adult' cordial. Zero-alcohol wines, beers and even spirits from boutique distilleries are also becoming increasingly popular.

One thing to consider is whether you want to drink non-alcoholic versions of your former go-to drinks. For some, the visual association can be triggering. Personally, I prefer to steer clear of anything that resembles my old drinking habits, just to be safe. It's all about knowing yourself and your triggers.

What do I do at 'that time of day'?

The routine and ritual of drinking can be one of the hardest things to break. How will you fill the time you'd normally spend with a glass in hand?

I like to focus on the positive aspects of being alcohol-free during my former 'witching hour'. Isn't it wonderful to know that if one of my children needs to be driven somewhere unexpectedly, even to the hospital emergency room, I can do so without hesitation because I haven't been drinking? Or that I have the energy to play with the dog, fold laundry or go for a family walk instead of being glued to the couch, nodding off after a few glasses of wine?

When on vacation, we can spontaneously take the kids out for an evening ice cream or a sunset beach stroll because we're not tied to a 5 p.m. 'drinkies' ritual.

The key is to establish a new routine. Find an alcohol-free beverage you enjoy. Look for the benefits in every moment of clarity and presence. Consciously appreciate your newfound freedom, and those positive associations will start to rewire your brain.

What do I do at social occasions when everyone else is drinking?

Navigating social situations can be tricky, especially when alcohol is a central part of the culture. The simplest solution is to always have a drink in hand – just make sure it's a non-alcoholic one! Bring a special mocktail or non-alcoholic boutique craft brewery treat to sip on. In case you still feel like you're missing out, think of a rare treat you could allow yourself – a new outfit, a salon treatment, a movie you've been wanting to see, a wickedly indulgent meal you don't normally partake in – and perhaps have that as a treat or reward for successfully not drinking in a difficult environment. Clearly, this can't be every and any time you face this scenario, as you'll then just be replacing one bad habit with another! But being mindful and overcoming the sense of 'missing out' by giving yourself something you value – an early night, a soak in a bath, some 'me-time' or other self-care activity that doesn't happen as much as you might like it to – is a good goal.

When at a social occasion, focus on really connecting with people and being present in the moment. Engage in meaningful conversations. Ask people questions and explore what makes them tick. People can be fascinating, if you see behind the facade. And remember, you're not missing out – you're gaining the ability to fully experience and remember the event.

You might even find that not drinking gives you a newfound superpower: the ability to observe the effects of alcohol on others from a sober perspective. Cherish your clear head and enjoy the authentic interactions.

What do I say when people ask why I'm not drinking?

This can be a delicate situation, and there's no one-size-fits-all response. Some people prefer to be direct and honest, sharing that they've decided to 'quit for health reasons' or because they 'didn't like how alcohol made me feel'. Others opt for a simpler 'I'm on a health kick' or 'I'm the designated driver tonight'.

Remember, you don't owe anyone a detailed explanation. It's your body and your choice. Find a response that feels authentic and comfortable to you and practise it so you're prepared when the question arises.

Here are some options to get you started:

- I'm taking a break from alcohol.

- I'm trying out a new fitness routine and cutting back on alcohol is part of it.

- I'm trying to save some money, so I'm cutting back on drinking.

- Alcohol tends to give me headaches, so I'm avoiding it tonight.

- I'm exploring different drink options and trying to expand my palate.

- I've realised I feel better overall when I don't drink.

- I'm taking part in a challenge to see how long I can go without alcohol.

- I'm choosing to be more mindful about what I consume, and tonight it's just not alcohol.

- I'm trying out being alcohol-free as an experiment to see how it impacts my life.

- I'm focusing on my mental wellbeing and cutting back on alcohol is part of that.

- I've decided to cut out alcohol for a while to see how it affects my sleep.

- I'm finding other ways to relax and unwind that don't involve alcohol.

- I simply don't feel like drinking tonight, and that's okay.

- I'm supporting a friend who's given up drinking.

- I'm avoiding alcohol to support a family member who's also not drinking.

- I've found that I'm more productive and focused without alcohol in my system.

- I've discovered some delicious non-alcoholic drinks I want to try instead.

- I'm participating in a 'dry month' challenge to reset my relationship with alcohol.

- I'm embracing alcohol-free as a lifestyle choice and feeling great about it.

- I've realised that I don't need alcohol to have a good time.

You know, sometimes we can even come up with hilarious responses, especially if we're the type who enjoys poking fun at ourselves. I'm sure you can think of a few! But let's be real — as funny as they are, they're not exactly boosting our self-esteem, are they? I've had mentors call me out on those self-deprecating jokes before. They're like little 'put-downs', and when we're all about building confidence and avoiding feeling bad about ourselves, that's not the vibe we want. So, let's find that sweet spot between not taking ourselves too seriously and not putting ourselves down. Believe me, a confident attitude can work wonders – people sometimes even think we've got superpowers! So, if you've got to 'fake it till you make it', do that!

How do I handle cravings?

Cravings are a normal part of the recovery process, but they don't have to control you. Science offers some powerful tools for managing these urges:

- **Understand the neurobiology of cravings.** Your brain has been wired to associate alcohol with reward. When you crave a drink, it's not a moral failing – it's your brain doing what it's been trained to do. Knowing this can help you depersonalise the experience.

- **Remember that cravings are time-limited.** They may feel overwhelming in the moment, but they will pass. Ride the wave and know that relief is on the other side.

- **Practice mindfulness.** Mindfulness techniques like deep breathing and staying present can help you tolerate the discomfort of cravings without acting on them.

- **Know your triggers.** Certain people, places or emotions may spark a craving. Identifying these triggers can help you anticipate and avoid or navigate them.

- **Get moving.** Exercise has been shown to reduce alcohol cravings. Even a quick walk or a few minutes of stretching can make a difference.

- **Distract yourself.** When a craving hits, shift your focus to something else. Engage in an activity that requires your full attention, like a puzzle, a craft project or a favourite hobby.

- **Lean on your support system.** Don't hesitate to reach out to a trusted friend, family member or support group when you're struggling. Sometimes just voicing the craving out loud can lessen its power.

What are the best ways to fill time previously spent drinking? How do I address fears of being bored or lonely if not drinking?

This is the time to get creative, adopt a 'growth mindset' and explore ideas far and wide to find a new or several new interests that excite you. It might be necessary to try any number of different hobbies or activities to find one that 'fits', and if that's the case, so be it. Here's a list to get you thinking:

- **Sports, outdoors, physical and exercise**

    o   Fishing: Ocean, river, or beach

    o   Birdwatching: Coastal or inland

    o   Fitness activities: Jogging, cycling, swimming, fitness classes, attending a gym

    o   Group sports: Volleyball, soccer or football, netball, hockey and the like

    o   Geocaching: Treasure hunts using GPS coordinates

    o   Metal detecting: Searching for buried treasure or artefacts

    o   Hiking or nature walks: Exploring nature through hiking or leisurely walks

    o   Yoga and meditation: Attend guided classes

    o   Martial arts: Tae kwon do, judo, karate, tai chi

    o   Scuba diving: Off the beach or a boat

    o   Cycling: Road cycling or mountain biking

    o   Fencing: A dynamic and fast paced sport

    o   Axe throwing: Throwing axes at targets – a thrilling and unconventional hobby o   Archery: Promotes focus, discipline and physical coordination

o   Rock climbing: Indoor or outdoor rock walls

o   Roller or ice skating: But be careful and don't break your arm like I did!

o   Lawn bowls: A strategic and social sport of precision, strategy and camaraderie

- **Arts and crafts**

    o   Painting and drawing: Watercolours, acrylics or oils, and pencils or charcoal

    o   Knitting or crocheting: Create clothing, scarves, hats or blankets

    o   DIY candle making: Customise scents, colours and shapes

    o   Sculpting with clay: Tactile satisfaction and creativity

    o   Embroidery: Meditative and visually rewarding

    o   Jewellery making: Personal expression and creativity

    o   Paper crafts: Origami, scrapbooking or card-making

    o   DIY home decor: Upcycling old furniture, creating wall art or making decorative items

    o   Macramé: Knotting techniques to create plant hangers, wall hangings and more

    o   Pottery: Both therapeutic and rewarding

    o   Cross-stitching: A blend of creativity and mindfulness

o DIY soap making: Using natural ingredients and essential oils for home or gifts

o Woodworking: Create shelves, cutting boards or birdhouses for enjoyment and use

o DIY bath bombs: A relaxing and indulgent experience

o Photography: Digital or film

- **Hobbies**

    o Jigsaw puzzles: Relaxing and absorbing

    o Sewing: Practical and enjoyable

    o Gardening: Cultivating plants, flowers or vegetables in a garden or containers

    o Joining a gardening club: Connect with fellow gardening enthusiasts

    o Cooking or baking: Rewarding, enjoyable and healthy

    o Reading: Get lost in a good book to escape from everyday stress

    o Writing: Journalling, creative writing or blogging – writing can be a cathartic and fulfilling hobby

    o Playing a musical instrument: Challenging, rewarding and a means of self-expression

    o Learning a new language: Expand cultural horizons and cognitive abilities

    o Board games: Social interaction and entertainment with friends and family

    o Model building: Airplanes, cars or ships, Warhammer, dioramas, railways o Calligraphy: Artistic expression through elegant handwriting

o Astrophotography: Capturing images of celestial objects and night skies with a camera

o Genealogy: Researching family history and tracing ancestry

o Beekeeping: Fosters a deeper understanding of ecosystems and agriculture – and gives honey!

o Pottery wheel throwing: Hands-on artistic expression and craftsmanship

o Soapstone carving: A tactile and creative outlet

o Shell collecting: Exploring beaches and shorelines to collect and identify items

- **Other**

  o Volunteering: Not only helps others but also provides a sense of purpose and fulfilment

  o Becoming a Scout leader: Mentor and guide youth

  o Acting classes: Opportunity for self-expression, creativity and personal development

  o Singing classes: Develop vocal skills, improve musicality and gain confidence

  o Joining a choir: Gain a sense of belonging and joy through shared musical experiences

  o Starting a walking club: Enjoy the benefits of physical activity and social connection

  o Starting a reading or book club: Foster a love of reading and intellectual exchange o Starting a gardening club: Enjoy the fruits of your labour and the beauty of nature all in one activity

o Backyard chicken keeping: Care, company and fresh eggs!

o Native animal care and rescue: Play a vital role in protecting and preserving local wildlife

A proviso: Depending upon where you are in the world, some groups and clubs may have a strong culture of – you guessed it! – drinking after activity sessions. Get all the details and attend complimentary trial sessions to see what the culture is in the group or club you're exploring. You don't want to be jumping from the frying pan into the fire!

Keep searching until you find something or some things that get you so excited and enthusiastic that it's what you want to spend every spare minute doing. When the desire to engage in this activity is so strong that it consumes your mind, endeavour to make it become your hobby – your new habit – above and beyond any unhealthy and damaging habit (or habits).

How do I manage insomnia or sleep issues after quitting alcohol?

It's common to experience sleep disturbances when you first quit drinking. Alcohol may have helped you fall asleep initially, but as we noted in Chapter 1 it actually disrupts sleep later in the night, leading to poorer sleep quality overall.

As your body adjusts to life without alcohol, you may experience insomnia or vivid dreams. This is normal and will improve with time. In the meantime, focus on good sleep hygiene:

- Stick to a consistent sleep schedule, even on weekends.

- Create a relaxing bedtime routine, like reading or taking a warm bath.

- Keep your bedroom cool, dark and quiet.

- Avoid screens for at least an hour before bed.

- Exercise regularly, but not too close to bedtime.

If sleep problems persist, don't hesitate to talk to your doctor. They will be the one to help rule out any underlying issues and suggest additional strategies for getting your rest back on track.

How do I go about managing relationships with people who still drink?

You'll likely predict what we'll offer here. If the people you class as friends value your relationship, they will accept and respect that you now choose not to drink. This is one hundred percent a real scenario for us. Men have a beer together – even with their dads, in fact. Women also have those drinking friends – sometimes their mum – who they drink Champagne with. We diffuse any difficulty with these scenarios by being 'as much fun without the alcohol as we might have once been with it'! This approach is part of the process. If you're not necessarily relaxed and sociable without an alcoholic drink, then it's off to the personal coach and personal development books for you – to work on self-love, self-esteem and other social skills that stem from valuing yourself. Hiding behind a veil of alcohol is never going to develop that side of a person's personality. You'll find good people will love you for 'you', so do the work on yourself to love and value who you are and what you bring to your friendships – and the world at large.

What else do I need to consider?

As you navigate this new chapter of your life, be sure to prioritise self-care. Dealing with emotions like guilt, shame or anxiety is a normal part of the process. Be patient and compassionate with yourself. The world is changing, and by being part of a new paradigm – one where alcohol-free is a valid option – you get to be part of the change and lead the way!

Building a strong support network is crucial. Surround yourself with people who understand and encourage your choice to be a non-drinker.

This might mean joining a support group, working with a therapist or leaning on loved ones who respect your decision.

Stay engaged and excited about your alcohol-free life by trying new hobbies, taking on challenges and celebrating each milestone along the way. The more you fill your life with meaning and purpose, the easier it will be to maintain your alcohol-free lifestyle.

And remember, if you do slip up, it doesn't negate all your progress. Each day is a new opportunity to recommit to your goals and your health. Learn from any setbacks and keep moving forward.

As you move forward, remember that every step, no matter how small, is a step in the right direction. Celebrate your courage, your determination and your commitment to a brighter future. And when challenges arise, as they inevitably will, lean on the support of those who believe in you and in the incredible potential that lies ahead.

The journey ahead may not always be easy, but it will be worth it. By taking things one day at a time and staying connected to your reasons for quitting, you'll build a fulfilling life free from alcohol's grip. And who knows – your story may just inspire someone else to do the same.

As you walk this transformative journey, remember that you have the strength, resilience and wisdom within you to overcome any challenges that arise. Trust in the process, stay committed to your goals and celebrate every victory along the way. By embracing this new chapter and all the possibilities it holds, you'll discover a life filled with greater clarity, connection and joy than you ever thought possible. The world needs more trailblazers like you, leading the way and showing others that a fulfilling, alcohol-free life is not only possible but truly rewarding. So, go forth with confidence, knowing that you're part of a growing movement of individuals who are redefining their relationship with alcohol and creating a brighter future for themselves and those around them. Here's to your incredible journey ahead!

Chapter 6:

Putting It Into Practice (Your Turn!)

Congratulations on making it as far as this! You've absorbed a wealth of information about alcohol, its effects and the various approaches to quitting drinking. Now it's time to put that knowledge into action and create a personalised plan for achieving a future where you're in control of your drinking decisions.

In this chapter, we'll provide prompts, structure, suggestions and resources to help you craft a step-by-step road map to success. By the end, you'll have a practical, tailored plan that you can start implementing right away.

Time to Grab a Notebook or Journal and Make a Plan!

Consider purchasing a special lined journal with an attractive cover and a pen that feels good in your hand. This isn't a punishment for past behaviour, but a tool for creating a bright and exciting new future. Treat it as a fresh opportunity to invest in yourself and your wellbeing.

Note: A companion workbook will be available for purchase alongside this book in the near future. Keep an eye out for its release!

Crafting Your Personalised Plan

Step 1: Addressing Reality

In Chapter 5, we asked lots of thought-provoking questions and looked at the reality that if you consider the facts as honestly as possible, you have three main options to choose from:

- Keep drinking but attempt to cut back and have greater control.

- Quit drinking entirely.

- Quit drinking for a set period of time.

Once you've made your choice, you need to not only take action but also manage that decision for the long term – which can be just as challenging as making the initial decision.

Let's get started with personalising your plan:

- Reflect on your answers to the questions from the 'Realisation That There is a Problem' section in Chapter 5. Do you see a problem emerging?

- Consider the 'Information Gathering, Then Decision Time and Action Time' section. Do you feel you have enough information to move forward? If not, where can you find the additional knowledge you need?

- What do you plan to do? Will you keep drinking but try to cut back, quit entirely or quit for a set period? Write down your decision and the date.

- Do you agree it's action time? Where do you want to be this time next year? More importantly, if you avoid making a decision and taking action now, where might you be in a year's time?

Having made your decision and committed to taking action, it's time to address the 'Managing the Decision Long Term' portion of Chapter 5. Don't worry about tackling everything at once – we'll break it down step by step. For now, just start brainstorming ideas for how you might approach the various challenges that may arise as you maintain your new lifestyle.

Step 2: A New Daily Habit – A Healthy Life Ritual

Firstly, commit to checking in with this plan daily. Make it part of your morning ritual. It's all about forming a new, positive habit!

Understanding the Difference Between a Routine and a Ritual

While routines focus on practical tasks and efficiency (brushing teeth, getting dressed, etc.), rituals are more about symbolism, meaning and intentionality (meditation, reviewing goals, practicing gratitude).

In short, routines largely look after our physical needs and responsibilities, while rituals nurture our emotional and mental wellbeing.

As one of my coaches wisely said, 'I do what is in my best interest before I do what I feel like'. This mantra aligns perfectly with what we're trying to achieve here. Carefully chosen rituals can help us focus on what's truly good for us, even when our immediate desires might pull us in a different direction.

Examples of Morning Rituals to Consider

- **Meditation:** Start your day with a few minutes of meditation to centre yourself and set a positive tone. Regular meditation has been shown to reduce stress and anxiety by shrinking the amygdala, the brain's 'fear centre'.

- **Gratitude practice:** Take a moment to reflect on what you're grateful for, either by writing in a journal or simply acknowledging these things mentally. Focusing on gratitude activates the brain's reward and pleasure centres, improving overall mood and wellbeing.

- **Stretching or yoga:** Engage in gentle stretching or a short yoga session to wake up your body and increase flexibility and energy. These practices promote mindfulness and resilience by encouraging awareness of the mind–body connection.

- **Reading or affirmations:** Spend some time reading an inspiring book or reciting positive affirmations. Exposing yourself to uplifting content helps shift your mindset from negative to positive, fostering a more resilient and optimistic outlook.

- **Nature connection:** Take a short walk outside, spend time in a garden or simply sit by a window and appreciate the natural world. Connecting with nature, even briefly, has been shown to reduce stress, improve mood and enhance overall wellbeing.

- **Journalling:** Write down your thoughts, goals or intentions for the day. Journalling can be a powerful tool for managing stress, increasing self-awareness and promoting mental, emotional and even physical health.

- **Visualisation:** Picture yourself achieving your goals and envisage a successful day ahead. Visualisation activates the same brain regions as actually performing the visualised activity, increasing the likelihood of real-world success.

While you may not have time for all of these rituals every day, choose a few that resonate with you and commit to incorporating them into your morning routine. Remember, consistency is key – aim to engage in your chosen rituals daily, but don't beat yourself up if you miss a day. Just get back on track as soon as possible.

A Recommended Morning Ritual

If you're not sure where to start, here's a simple morning ritual to try:

1. Read your plan.

2. Write down three things you're grateful for.

3. Write down three things you're excited about.

4. Do a five-minute (minimum) meditation.

5. Do a five-minute (minimum) visualisation exercise.

A Recommended Evening Ritual

1. Write down three things that went well today.

2. Write down one note to yourself about what you can improve on tomorrow.

3. Accept that today went how today went, knowing you did the best you could today.

4. A meditation before going to sleep is calming and soothing and can promote better sleep quality.

Step 3: What's Your 'Why'?

After setting up your morning ritual in your notebook or the companion workbook, the next step is to review your 'why' – your reasons for wanting to change your relationship with alcohol.

If needed, revisit Chapter 3, where we explored four main reasons people choose to quit drinking:

- to live longer

- to live a healthier life

- to set a good example for loved ones and those you influence

- to have better relationships with loved ones

Your 'why' might encompass all of these reasons, and that's great! The more compelling your 'why', the more motivated you'll be to stick to your plan.

This is also the place to record your vision of success. What will your life look like when you've achieved your goal of quitting drinking or cutting back? Use lots of detail and engage all your senses. If you enjoy creating vision boards, this is the perfect opportunity to make one.

The Power of Writing in the Present Tense

When recording your vision of success, write as though you're already living it. This is where visualisation can be not only enjoyable but also incredibly powerful. If you can tap into that little tingle of excitement as you imagine yourself in your successful future (happily not drinking while everyone around you is, exuding confidence and joy, pursuing your dreams with a clear head and healthy body), you've struck gold. Being able to close your eyes and conjure up that feeling whenever you need a boost will be invaluable on the tougher days.

Research supports the effectiveness of this technique, known as 'future self journalling' or 'future pacing'. Studies show that vividly imagining your future self can help you make better decisions in the present, reduce impulsivity and increase your motivation to achieve long-term goals (Daniel et al., 2013).

So, don't be shy – dream big, and write it all down in glorious detail!

Step 4: Contemplate the Facts, Then Let Them Go

Re-read Chapter 2: 'Why Do People Develop Issues With Alcohol?' Find a quiet place to sit and reflect on which factors from this chapter might be relevant to your situation.

However, you're not going to dwell on these factors by writing them down in your journal. The goal is to acknowledge and accept what has been, then release it and move forward. If you feel compelled to write these things down, do so on a separate piece of paper. Read it over one last time, then ceremoniously (and safely!) burn the paper, symbolically letting go of the past.

This step is important because we want to recognise that there are logical, scientific reasons why we've ended up struggling with alcohol. It's not because we're weak or morally flawed. Our biology, genes, environment or a combination of these factors have simply stacked the deck against us.

By acknowledging this truth, we can release any shame or self-blame we might be harbouring and move forward with compassion for ourselves. We can make conscious choices that empower us to take control of our relationship with alcohol, armed with the knowledge that we're not alone in this struggle.

Step 5: Which Approach Suits You?

Revisit Chapter 4. Notice which approaches resonate with you and align with your values.

For instance, if you prioritise holistic health, you might be drawn to the comprehensive lifestyle changes outlined in Option 8. (In fact, we recommend everyone consider incorporating these changes, regardless of what other approaches they choose!)

If you and your healthcare provider determine that MAT is appropriate for your situation, learn all you can about this option. Remember, knowledge is power. The more informed and proactive you are, the better equipped you'll be to make decisions that support your long-term success.

It's important to note that what works for one person might not work for another. Some may find success with a self-guided approach and minimal support, while others might require the structure and community of a formal rehabilitation programme. Trust your instincts and be honest about what level of support you need.

If you're seeking professional help and feel like you're not being heard or taken seriously, don't hesitate to seek a second opinion. Keep advocating for yourself until you find the right fit. Your wellbeing is worth it!

In your journal or the companion workbook, write down the quit-drinking approaches and support methods that appeal to you and are feasible given your circumstances.

Decide which option(s) you'll pursue and identify your next steps. Create a timeline for getting started and set some milestones to help you stay on track.

Sample Quit-Drinking Plan

1. I will schedule a health assessment with my primary care provider and discuss my plans with them.

2. I will quit drinking for 12 months and reassess after that time.

3. To ensure I have emotional support and accountability, I will find a coach, therapist or counsellor experienced in helping people navigate alcohol dependence and untangle any emotional and mental health issues.

4. My nutrition plan to support optimal health during this transition includes:

    o following my healthcare provider's recommendations to address any nutrient deficiencies

    o engaging in regular exercise, such as daily walks, swimming or dancing

    o staying hydrated by drinking plenty of water and limiting caffeine intake

    o choosing whole foods over processed options whenever possible

5. To prioritise restful sleep, I will:

o   stick to a consistent sleep schedule

o   keep my bedroom dark, quiet and cool

o   avoid eating within two hours of bedtime

o   disconnect from screens at least an hour before sleep

6. I will explore alcohol-free beverage options:

o   for evenings when I would typically drink

o   to enjoy while cooking, when cravings often strike

o   to order when out with friends or at social events

Note: Be mindful of substituting alcohol with high-sugar or heavily processed drinks, as these can pose their own health challenges. Aim for mostly water, herbal tea and other natural, low-sugar options.

7. To keep my mind and hands occupied during times I might normally drink, I will:

o   explore a new hobby or revisit an old one that brings me joy

o   engage in activities that promote physical, mental and emotional wellbeing

o   seek out social connections and support through clubs, classes or volunteer work

Write down a list of half a dozen or so hobbies and activities that excite you. You can refer to the extensive list in Chapter 5. The key is to find something so engaging and rewarding that it naturally becomes your go-to activity, replacing any unhealthy habits you're trying to leave behind.

8. When people ask why I'm not drinking, I will say:

> o *From Chapter 5, choose three options that will roll off your tongue easily (once you've practised them a bit!). Or try out some of your own, researching for more inspiration online if you'd like.*

Remember, the goal is to build a life so full of meaning and joy that alcohol loses its appeal. By taking the time to thoughtfully craft your personalised plan, you're laying the foundation for lasting success.

Step 6: Managing FOMO (Fear of Missing Out)

In today's hyper-connected world, it's easy to fall into the trap of comparing our lives to others, especially on social media. This can lead to FOMO, or the fear of missing out, which is the pervasive apprehension that others might be having rewarding experiences from which one is absent.

Research shows that FOMO is linked to lower life satisfaction, mood and self-esteem. It can also lead to problematic social media use and a distorted perception of reality (Elhai et al., 2016; Oberst et al., 2017; Przybylski et al., 2013). For those pursuing an alcohol-free lifestyle, FOMO can be a significant obstacle, as social drinking is often portrayed as the norm and a prerequisite for having fun.

To manage FOMO during your journey:

- **Reframe your perspective.** Instead of focusing on what you might be missing out on, shift your attention to what you're gaining by choosing an alcohol-free life. Remind yourself of your 'why' and the future you're working towards.

- **Practise gratitude.** Regularly take time to appreciate the good things in your life. Keeping a gratitude journal can help you maintain a positive outlook and reduce the impact of FOMO.

- **Curate your social media feed.** Unfollow or mute accounts that trigger your FOMO or glamorise drinking. Instead, seek out inspirational content that aligns with your goals and values.

- **Engage in meaningful activities.** Pursue hobbies, interests and social connections that bring you genuine fulfilment. When you're living a life aligned with your values, FOMO loses its power.

- **Play the tape forward.** When FOMO strikes, imagine yourself in the future, having achieved your goals and living your best life. Contrast that with the temporary discomfort of missing out on a drinking-centred event.

Remember, FOMO is a normal human experience, but it doesn't have to control your actions. By staying grounded in your 'why', practising mindfulness and focusing on your own path, you can overcome FOMO and stay committed to your alcohol-free journey.

Still Got Doubts? Addressing Resistance to Change

It's natural to have doubts or feel resistant to change. These feelings are a normal part of the process and don't mean you're destined to fail. To work through any lingering doubts, try this exercise:

1. Write down all the reasons you think this won't work for you. Be honest and thorough, listing every objection that comes to mind.

2. Take a deep breath and sit with each reason for a moment. Ask yourself:

   o Is this an excuse or a legitimate concern?

   o Have I fully committed to making this change, or am I still undecided?

   o Is my 'why' strong enough to help me overcome this obstacle?

3. For each reason that feels like an excuse, acknowledge it as such and let it go. Remind yourself that you're stronger than

your excuses and that you have the power to choose a different path.

4. For any legitimate concerns, brainstorm solutions or identify the support you need to address them. This might involve reaching out to professionals, leaning on your support network or developing new coping strategies.

5. If you find that your commitment to change is wavering, revisit your 'why' and the vision of your future self. Reconnect with the reasons you embarked on this journey in the first place and let that motivation reignite your determination.

Remember, change is rarely easy, but it is always possible. By acknowledging and working through your doubts, you demonstrate incredible strength and resilience. Be patient and compassionate with yourself, and trust that every step forward, no matter how small, is a victory worth celebrating.

Keys to Success

Making a major lifestyle change like this is no small feat. To stay committed and motivated, keep these three things in mind:

- Always remember your 'why':

    o Keep your reasons for quitting front and centre.

    o Write them down and refer to them often, especially when temptation strikes.

- Fully embrace the benefits of your new lifestyle:

    o Celebrate your clear head, improved sleep, increased energy and enhanced presence.

- Appreciate how much easier it is to work towards your goals without alcohol holding you back.

- When an urge arises, play the tape forward:

  - Allow yourself to briefly remember the worst parts of drinking – the hangovers, the shame, the lost time.

  - Contrast that with all you've gained in adopting an alcohol-free lifestyle.

Define what success looks like for you and keep that vision in mind. Whether it's improved relationships, better health, career progression or personal growth, keeping your eyes on the prize will help you stay the course.

Celebrate!

Congratulations on taking the time to create your personalised plan for transforming your relationship with alcohol. By reflecting on your motivations, considering various approaches and outlining specific strategies for self-care and building a fulfilling life, you've set yourself up for success.

Remember, this plan is a living document – a road map that can evolve as you learn and grow. Embrace the flexibility to adjust your course as needed while staying true to your ultimate goal of reclaiming control over your drinking decisions.

As you start this journey, be patient and compassionate with yourself. Change takes time, and there may be setbacks along the way. When challenges arise, refer back to your plan and lean on the support systems you've put in place. Celebrate your progress, no matter how small, and keep your eyes on the bright future you're creating.

The path to a healthier, more balanced life is rarely a straight line. It's a winding road with ups and downs, triumphs and obstacles. But with each step forward, you'll grow stronger, more resilient and more confident in your ability to navigate whatever comes your way.

So, take a deep breath, trust in the process and have faith in yourself. You've got this! Your commitment to personal growth and wellbeing is a powerful force that will guide you through the toughest times and lead you to a life of greater joy, purpose and fulfilment.

As you move forward, remember that you're not alone. Countless others have walked this path before you and have found the strength to transform their lives. Draw inspiration from their stories and know that you, too, have the power to create lasting, positive change.

Your journey begins here, with this plan as your compass. Embrace the adventure, stay curious and never stop learning. The rewards of a life free from alcohol's grip are immeasurable – improved health, stronger relationships, clearer thinking and a renewed sense of purpose and possibility.

So here's to you, your courage and the incredible future you're creating, one day at a time. May your journey be filled with discovery, growth and the unwavering knowledge that you are capable of achieving extraordinary things.

Wishing you success and joy in your planning!

Conclusion

There's no sugar-coating it: breaking free from an unhealthy relationship with alcohol is a challenging journey. For some of us, moderation simply isn't an option. When faced with this situation, we have two choices: take control of our relationship with alcohol and embrace a longer, more vibrant life, or continue to let alcohol dictate our choices and limit our potential.

But here's the good news: it is possible to leave this toxic relationship behind. Throughout this book, we've armed you with the knowledge and tools you need to make a lasting change.

We've examined the pros and cons of alcohol, both as a substance and as a beverage. We've explored the internal and external factors that can lead to alcohol dependence, providing a scientific foundation for understanding your own relationship with drinking.

We've also reviewed the most widely accepted methods for quitting alcohol, drawing from a range of approaches to help you find the path that aligns with your unique needs and values.

Ultimately, this journey is about empowering you to make informed decisions about your health and well-being. By guiding you through a three-step process, we've helped you transform knowledge into action:

1. **Realisation that there is a problem:** By honestly assessing your drinking habits and their impact on your life, you've taken the crucial first step towards change.

2. **Information gathering, decision time and action time:** Armed with a comprehensive understanding of alcohol and its effects, you've evaluated your options and made a clear decision about your next steps. Whether you've chosen to quit

entirely, take a break, or pursue moderation, you've developed a personalised action plan to guide your journey.

3. **Managing the decision long term:** Quitting drinking is not a one-time event, but a lifelong commitment. By anticipating challenges, building a strong support network and prioritising self-care, you've laid the foundation for lasting success.

As you embark on this transformative journey, remember that you're not alone. Countless individuals have walked this path before you, and their stories serve as a testament to the incredible resilience and strength of the human spirit.

Embrace the discomfort of change, knowing that it's a sign of growth. Celebrate each milestone, no matter how small, and be kind to yourself when faced with setbacks. Most importantly, never lose sight of your 'why' – the profound reasons that motivated you to make this life-altering decision.

Breaking free from alcohol's grip is not about deprivation or punishment. It's about liberation, self-discovery and reclaiming your right to a life unburdened by addiction. It's about waking up each day with a clear mind, a healthier body and a renewed sense of purpose.

By reading this book and committing to change, you've already taken a monumental step towards a brighter future. You've acknowledged that your relationship with alcohol no longer serves you, and you've made the courageous choice to prioritise your well-being.

As you continue on this path, remember that progress is rarely linear. There will be challenges and triumphs, moments of doubt and flashes of profound clarity. Through it all, trust in your inherent strength and resilience. Lean on the support of loved ones, and don't hesitate to seek professional guidance when needed.

Your journey towards freedom from alcohol is a powerful testament to your commitment to living life on your own terms. Embrace this opportunity to rediscover yourself, to explore new passions and possibilities and to cultivate a deep sense of self-love and acceptance.

You have the power within you to rewrite your story and create a future filled with joy, purpose and boundless potential. Hold tight to your dreams, and trust in the transformative power of this journey.

One day at a time, one choice at a time, you are building a life beyond your wildest dreams – a life in which you are the author, the hero, and the master of your own destiny.

So, take a deep breath, square your shoulders and step forward with confidence. Your most vibrant, fulfilling life awaits.

References

Abrahao, K. P., Salinas, A. G., & Lovinger, D. M. (2017). Alcohol and the brain: Neuronal molecular targets, synapses, and circuits. *Neuron*, *96*(6), 1223–1238. https://doi.org/10.1016/j.neuron.2017.10.032

Adriaanse, M. A., Gollwitzer, P. M., De Ridder, D. T. D., de Wit, J. B. F., & Kroese, F. M. (2011). Breaking habits with implementation intentions: A test of underlying processes. *Personality and Social Psychology Bulletin*, *37*(4), 502–513. https://doi.org/10.1177/0146167211399102

Afifi, T. O., Enns, M. W., Cox, B. J., Asmundson, G. J., Stein, M. B., & Sareen, J. (2008). Population attributable fractions of psychiatric disorders and suicide ideation and tries associated with adverse childhood experiences. *American Journal of Public Health*, *98*(5), 946-952. https://doi.org/10.2105/AJPH.2007.120253

Audiffren, M., André, N., & Baumeister, R. F. (2022). Training willpower: Reducing costs and valuing effort. *Frontiers in Neuroscience, 16*. https://doi.org/10.3389/fnins.2022.699817

Becker, H. C. (2012). Effects of alcohol dependence and withdrawal on stress responsiveness and alcohol consumption. *Alcohol Research: Current Reviews, 34*(4), 448–458. https://www.ncbi.nlm.nih.gov/pmc/articles/PMC3860383/

Brady, K. T., & Back, S. E. (2012). Childhood trauma, posttraumatic stress disorder, and alcohol dependence. *Alcohol Research: Current Reviews, 34*(4), 408–413. https://www.ncbi.nlm.nih.gov/pmc/articles/PMC3860395/

Burri, A., Maercker, A., Krammer, S., & Simmen-Janevska, K. (2013). Childhood trauma and PTSD symptoms increase the risk of cognitive impairment in a sample of former indentured child laborers in old age. *PLoS ONE*, *8*(2), e57826. https://doi.org/10.1371/journal.pone.0057826

Carrigan, M. A., Uryasev, O., Frye, C. B., Eckman, B. L., Myers, C. R., Hurley, T. D., & Benner, S. A. (2014). Hominids adapted to metabolize ethanol long before human-directed fermentation. *Proceedings of the National Academy of Sciences*, 112(2), 458–463. https://doi.org/10.1073/pnas.1404167111

Chiva-Blanch, G., & Badimon, L. (2019). Benefits and risks of moderate alcohol consumption on cardiovascular disease: Current findings and controversies. *Nutrients*, 12(1), 108. https://doi.org/10.3390/nu12010108

Church, D., Stapleton, P., Mollon, P., Feinstein, D., Boath, E., Mackay, D., & Sims, R. (2018). Guidelines for the treatment of PTSD using clinical EFT (emotional freedom techniques). *Healthcare*, 6(4). https://doi.org/10.3390/healthcare6040146

Colrain, I. M., Nicholas, C. L., & Baker, F. C. (2014). Alcohol and the sleeping brain. In E. V. Sullivan & A. Pfefferbaum (Eds.), *Handbook of Clinical Neurology*, *125*, 415–431. https://doi.org/10.1016/B978-0-444-62619-6.00024-0

Daniel, T. O., Stanton, C. M., & Epstein, L. H. (2013). The future is now: Reducing impulsivity and energy intake using episodic future thinking. *Psychological Science*, 24(11), 2339–2342. https://doi.org/10.1177/0956797613488780

Edenberg, H. (2013). Genetics of alcohol use disorders. In P. M. Miller (Ed.), *biological research on addiction: Comprehensive addictive behaviors and disorders*, Volume 2. Elsevier. https://doi.org/10.1016/C2011-0-07782-7

Elhai, J. D., Levine, J. C., Dvorak, R. D., & Hall, B. J. (2016). Fear of missing out, need for touch, anxiety and depression are related to problematic smartphone use. *Computers in Human Behavior*, 63,

509-516.
https://psycnet.apa.org/doi/10.1016/j.chb.2016.05.079

Gardner, B., Lally, P., & Wardle, J. (2012). Making health habitual: The psychology of 'habit-formation' and general practice. *British Journal of General Practice*, *62*(605), 664–666. https://doi.org/10.3399/bjgp12X659466

Greenberg, L. S. (2017). *Emotion-focused therapy*. American Psychological Association. https://doi.org/10.1037/15971-001

Higuchi, S., Matsushita, S., Muramatsu, T., Murayama, M., & Hayashida, M. (1996). Alcohol and aldehyde dehydrogenase genotypes and drinking behavior in Japanese. *Alcoholism: Clinical and Experimental Research*, *20*(3), 493–497. https://doi.org/10.1111/j.1530-0277.1996.tb01080.x

Hoyumpa, A. M. (1986). Mechanisms of vitamin deficiencies in alcoholism. *Alcoholism: Clinical and Experimental Research*, *10*(6), 573–581. https://doi.org/10.1111/j.1530-0277.1986.tb05147.x

Jemberie, W. B., Padyab, M., Snellman, F., & Lundgren, L. (2020). A multidimensional latent class analysis of harmful alcohol use among older adults: Subtypes within the Swedish Addiction Severity Index Registry. *Journal of Addiction Medicine*, *14*(4), e89–e99. https://doi.org/10.1097/adm.0000000000000636

Kesmodel, U., Wisborg, K., Olsen, S. F., Henrisksen, T. B., & Secher, N. J. (2002). Moderate alcohol intake in pregnancy and the risk of spontaneous abortion. *Alcohol and Alcoholism*, *37*(1), 87–92. https://doi.org/10.1093/alcalc/37.1.87

Kono, S., Ikeda, M., Tokudome, S., Nishizumi, M., & Kuratsune, M. (1986). Alcohol and mortality: A cohort study of male Japanese physicians. *International Journal of Epidemiology*, *15*(4), 527–532. https://doi.org/10.1093/ije/15.4.527

Kushner, M. G., Abrams, K., Thuras, P., Hanson, K. L., Brekke, M., & Sletten, S. (2005). Follow-up study of anxiety disorder and alcohol dependence in comorbid alcoholism treatment patients.

Alcoholism: Clinical & Experimental Research, 29(8), 1432–1443. https://doi.org/10.1097/01.alc.0000175072.17623.f8

Lookatch, S. J., Wimberly, A. S., & McKay, J. R. (2019). Effects of social support and 12-step involvement on recovery among people in continuing care for cocaine dependence. *Substance Use & Misuse, 54*(13), 2144–2155. https://doi.org/10.1080/10826084.2019.1638406

Maraboli, S. (2022, January 2). *Incredible change happens in your life when you decide to take control of what you do have power over instead of craving control over what you don't* [Image attached] [Status update]. Facebook. https://www.facebook.com/photo/?fbid=2821065447916136&set=a.690866084269427

McDonald, J. A., Goyal, A., & Terry, M. B. (2013). Alcohol intake and breast cancer risk: Weighing the overall evidence. *Current Breast Cancer Reports, 5*(3), 208–221. https://doi.org/10.1007/s12609-013-0114-z

Mehta, D., Klengel, T., Conneely, K. N., Smith, A. K., Altmann, A., Pace, T. W., Rex-Haffner, M., Loeschner, A., Gonik, M., Mercer, K. B., Bradley, B., Muller-Myhsok, B., Ressler, K. J., & Binder, E. B. (2013). Childhood maltreatment is associated with distinct genomic and epigenetic profiles in posttraumatic stress disorder. *Proceedings of the National Academy of Sciences, 110*(20), 8302–8307. https://doi.org/10.1073/pnas.1217750110

Mercille, J. (2017). Media coverage of alcohol issues: A critical political economy framework—A case study from Ireland. *International Journal of Environmental Research and Public Health, 14*(6), 650. https://doi.org/10.3390/ijerph14060650

Merikangas, K. R., Stevens, D., & Fenton, B. (1996). Comorbidity of alcoholism and anxiety disorders: The role of family studies. *Alcohol Health and Research World, 20*(2), 100–106. https://www.ncbi.nlm.nih.gov/pmc/articles/PMC6876502/

Miller, W. R., Walters, S. T., & Bennett, M. E. (2001). How effective is alcoholism treatment in the United States? *Journal of Studies on Alcohol,* *62*(2), 211–220. https://doi.org/10.15288/jsa.2001.62.211

Moos, R. H., & Moos, B. S. (2006). Participation in treatment and Alcoholics Anonymous: A 16-year follow-up of initially untreated individuals. *Journal of Clinical Psychology, 62*(6), 735–750. https://doi.org/10.1002/jclp.20259

Nemeroff, C. B. (2003). The role of GABA in the pathophysiology and treatment of anxiety disorders. *Psychopharmacology Bulletin,* 37(4), 133–146.

Nestor, J. (2020). *Breath: the new science of a lost art.* Riverhead Books.

NPR Staff. (2014, March 24). *With sobering science, doctor debunks 12-step recovery.* NPR. https://www.npr.org/2014/03/23/291405829/with-sobering-science-doctor-debunks-12-step-recovery

Oberst, U., Wegmann, E., Stodt, B., Brand, M., & Chamarro, A. (2017). Negative consequences from heavy social networking in adolescents: The mediating role of fear of missing out. *Journal of Adolescence,* *55,* 51-60. https://doi.org/10.1016/j.adolescence.2016.12.00

Oh, V. K. S., Sarwar, A., & Pervez, N. (2022). The study of mindfulness as an intervening factor for enhanced psychological well-being in building the level of resilience. Frontiers in Psychology, 13. https://doi.org/10.3389/fpsyg.2022.1056834

O'Leary, C. M., Taylor, C., Zubrick, S. R., Kurinczuk, J. J., & Bower, C. (2013). Prenatal alcohol exposure and educational achievement in children aged 8-9 years. *Pediatrics, 132*(2), e468-475. https://doi.org/10.1542/peds.2012-3002

Osna, N. A., Donohue, T. M., & Kharbanda, K. K. (2017). Alcoholic liver disease: Pathogenesis and current management. *Alcohol*

Research: Current Reviews, 38(2), 147–161. https://www.ncbi.nlm.nih.gov/pmc/articles/PMC5513682/

Palzes, V. A., Parthasarathy, S., Chi, F. W., Kline-Simon, A. H., Lu, Y., Weisner, C., Ross, T. B., Elson, J., & Sterling, S. A. (2020). Associations between psychiatric disorders and alcohol consumption levels in an adult primary care population. *Alcoholism: Clinical and Experimental Research, 44*(12), 2536–2544. https://doi.org/10.1111/acer.14477

Peppard, P. E., Austin, D., & Brown, R. L. (2007). Association of alcohol consumption and sleep disordered breathing in men and women. *Journal of Clinical Sleep Medicine, 3*(3), 265–270. https://www.ncbi.nlm.nih.gov/pmc/articles/PMC2564771/265-270.

Petti, S., & Scully, C. (2005). Alcohol consumption and oral cancer: a study in Italy. *British Journal of Cancer, 92*(5), 899–900.

Piano, M. R. (2017). Alcohol's effects on the cardiovascular system. *Alcohol Research: Current Reviews, 38*(2), 219–241. https://www.ncbi.nlm.nih.gov/pmc/articles/PMC5513687/

Przybylski, A. K., Murayama, K., DeHaan, C. R., & Gladwell, V. (2013). Motivational, emotional, and behavioral correlates of fear of missing out. *Computers in Human Behavior, 29*(4), 1841–1848https://doi.org/10.1016/j.chb.2013.02.014

Robertson, A. G., Easter, M. M., Lin, H., Frisman, L. K., Swanson, J. W., & Swartz, M. S. (2018). Medication-assisted treatment for alcohol-dependent adults with serious mental illness and criminal justice involvement: Effects on treatment utilization and outcomes. *American Journal of Psychiatry, 175*(7), 665–673. https://doi.org/10.1176/appi.ajp.2018.17060688

Sabia, S., Elbaz, A., Britton, A., Bell, S., Dugravot, A., Shipley, M., Kivimaki, M., & Singh-Manoux, A. (2014). Alcohol consumption and cognitive decline in early old age. *Neurology, 82*(4), 332–339. https://doi.org/10.1212/wnl.0000000000000063

Schuckit, M. A. (2009). An overview of genetic influences in alcoholism. *Journal of Substance Abuse Treatment, 36*(1), S5–14. https://pubmed.ncbi.nlm.nih.gov/19062348/

Schuckit, M. A., Tipp, J. E., Reich, T., Hesselbrock, v. M., & Bucholz, K. K. (2006). The histories of withdrawal convulsions and delirium tremens in 1648 alcohol dependent subjects. *Addiction, 90*(10), 1335–1347. https://doi.org/10.1046/j.1360-0443.1995.901013355.x

Scott, C., & Corbin, W. R. (2014). Influence of sensation seeking on response to alcohol versus placebo: Implications for the acquired preparedness model. *Journal of Studies on Alcohol and Drugs, 75*(1), 136–144. https://doi.org/10.1046/j.1360-0443.1995.901013355.x

Shin, S. H., Hong, H. G., & Jeon, S.-M. (2012). Personality and alcohol use: The role of impulsivity. *Addictive Behaviors, 37*(1), 102–107. https://doi.org/10.1016/j.addbeh.2011.09.006

Smith, R. J., & Laiks, L. S. (2018). Behavioral and neural mechanisms underlying habitual and compulsive drug seeking. *Progress in Neuro-Psychopharmacology and Biological Psychiatry, 87*, 11–21. https://doi.org/10.1016/j.pnpbp.2017.09.003

Sood, B., Delaney-Black, V., Covington, C., Nordstrom-Klee, B., Ager, J., Templin, T., Janisse, J., Martier, S., & Sokol, R. J. (2001). Prenatal alcohol exposure and childhood behavior at age 6 to 7 years: I. Dose-response effect. *Pediatrics, 108*(2), e34. https://doi.org/10.1542/peds.108.2.e34

Soundararajan, S., Narayanan, G., Agrawal, A., Prabhakaran, D., & Murthy, P. (2017). Relation between age at first alcohol drink & adult life drinking patterns in alcohol-dependent patients. *The Indian Journal of Medical Research, 146*(5), 606–611. https://doi.org/10.4103%2Fijmr.IJMR_1363_15

Stockwell, T., Zhao, J., Panwar, S., Roemer, A., Naimi, T., & Chikritzhs, T. (2016). Do "moderate" drinkers have reduced mortality risk? A systematic review and meta-analysis of alcohol consumption and all-cause mortality. *Journal of Studies on Alcohol and Drugs, 77*(2), 185–198. https://doi.org/10.15288/jsad.2016.77.185

Taillieu, T. L., Brownridge, D. A., Sareen, J., & Afifi, T. O. (2016). Childhood emotional maltreatment and mental disorders: Results from a nationally representative adult sample from the United States. *Child Abuse & Neglect, 59*, 1–12. https://doi.org/10.1016/j.chiabu.2016.07.005

Testino, G. (2011). The burden of cancer attributable to alcohol consumption. *Maedica, 6*(4), 313–320. https://www.ncbi.nlm.nih.gov/pmc/articles/PMC3391950/

Tezal, M., Grossi, S. G., Ho, A. W., & Genco, R. J. (2001). The effect of alcohol consumption on periodontal disease. *Journal of Periodontology, 72*(2), 183–189. https://doi.org/10.1902/jop.2001.72.2.183

Traversy, G., & Chaput, J.-P. (2018). Alcohol consumption and obesity: An update. *Current Obesity Reports, 4*(1), 122–130. https://doi.org/10.1007%2Fs13679-014-0129-4

Tyas, S. L. (2001). Alcohol use and the risk of developing Alzheimer's disease. *Alcohol Research & Health, 25*(4), 299–306. https://www.ncbi.nlm.nih.gov/pmc/articles/pmc6705707/

Wakabayashi, M., Sugiyama, Y., Takada, M., Kinjo, A., Iso, H., & Tabuchi, T. (2022). Loneliness and increased hazardous alcohol use: Data from a nationwide internet survey with 1-year follow-up. *International Journal of Environmental Research and Public Health, 19*(19), 12086. https://doi.org/10.3390/ijerph191912086

Walker, M. P. (2017). *Why we sleep: Unlocking the power of sleep and dreams.* Scribner.

Xie, L., Kang, H., Xu, Q., Chen, M. J., Liao, Y., Thiyagarajan, M., O'Donnell, J., Christensen, D. J., Nicholson, C., Iliff, J. J., Takano, T., Deane, R., & Nedergaard, M. (2013). Sleep drives metabolite clearance from the adult brain. *Science, 342*(6156), 373-7.

Zhang, C., Qing, N., & Zhang, S. (2021). The impact of leisure activities on the mental health of older adults: The mediating effect of social support and perceived stress. *Journal of Healthcare Engineering,* 2021, 6264447. https://doi.org/10.1155/2021/6264447

Printed in Great Britain
by Amazon

42812036R00089